Ouanassa Hamouda
Nabila Kalla
Ahlem Merzougui

Oral candidiasis in diabetics

Ouanassa Hamouda
Nabila Kalla
Ahlem Merzougui

Oral candidiasis in diabetics

ScienciaScripts

Imprint
Any brand names and product names mentioned in this book are subject to trademark, brand or patent protection and are trademarks or registered trademarks of their respective holders. The use of brand names, product names, common names, trade names, product descriptions etc. even without a particular marking in this work is in no way to be construed to mean that such names may be regarded as unrestricted in respect of trademark and brand protection legislation and could thus be used by anyone.

Cover image: www.ingimage.com

This book is a translation from the original published under ISBN 978-620-6-72826-9.

Publisher:
Sciencia Scripts
is a trademark of
Dodo Books Indian Ocean Ltd. and OmniScriptum S.R.L publishing group

120 High Road, East Finchley, London, N2 9ED, United Kingdom
Str. Armeneasca 28/1, office 1, Chisinau MD-2012, Republic of Moldova, Europe
Managing Directors: Ieva Konstantinova, Victoria Ursu
info@omniscriptum.com

Printed at: see last page
ISBN: 978-620-8-50918-7

TABLE OF CONTENTS

INTRODUCTION

In the 21st century, diabetes is becoming a global epidemic and one of the greatest emerging threats to public health, significantly patients' quality of life and longevity, as well as healthcare costs [1].

Diabetes mellitus is one of the most common endocrine disorders, signified by the presence of long-term hyperglycaemia [1].

There are two types of diabetes: type 1 diabetes is characterised by complete insulin deficiency due to the destruction of pancreatic beta cells, and type 2 diabetes by insulin resistance, which can eventually lead to hyperglycaemia [2].

Diabetes causes long-term complications such as retinopathy, neuropathy and nephropathy, generally accelerating macro- and micro-vascular changes [3].

In 2017, the global prevalence of diabetes adults (aged 20-79) was almost 425 million, and the World Health Organization and the International Diabetes Federation have predicted that the number of adults with diabetes worldwide will reach almost 629 million by 2045 [3].

Diabetes mellitus is the cause of many infectious symptoms and complications, such as dry mouth, taste disorders, oral candidiasis, rhinocerebral zygomycosis (mucormycosis), aspergillosis, geographic tongue, oral lichen planus, delayed healing, periodontal disease and gingivitis. Yeast infections are common in diabetic patients [2].

According to the American Diabetes Association, patients with diabetes suffer from a major problem of a weak immune system that hinders their ability to fight off intrusive micro-organisms, making them more prone to infections. Recovery time from infection or injury in people with diabetes is significantly prolonged compared to the healthy population and the relationship between diabetes and candidiasis has been extensively studied, particularly because of the increased susceptibility of diabetic patients to fungal infections compared to non-diabetic patients [2].

Oral candidiasis is one of the most common fungal infections affecting the oral mucosa [4].

Previous studies have shown that the saliva of people with diabetes contains a greater number of Candida colony-forming units than the saliva of healthy subjects. A higher incidence of Candida species is found in the oral cavity of the DM patient due to various factors such as reduced salivary flow rates, higher salivary glucose concentrations, reduced host defence system due reduced neutrophil activity and greater adherence of Candida species to oral epithelial cells [2].

A number of Candida species are usually found as harmless commensals in the digestive tract, oral cavity and genital region of healthy individuals, oral Candida (C) species include Candida albicans, Candida glabrata, Candida guillermondii, Candida krusei, Candida parapsilosis, Candida pseudotropicalis, Candida stellatoidea and Candida tropicalis [4,5].

Certain factors have a major influence on balance between host and yeast and have caused Candida to transition from commensal to pathogenic status and cause oral infection. These include reduced salivary flow, increased salivary glucose levels altered neutrophil acid candi activity [1].

The risk factors for oral candidiasis are complex, but we know that lesions on the tongue, smoking, alcohol consumption, wearing dentures, taking medication and immunosuppression such as diabetes are risk factors that clearly influence oral candidiasis [1].

Given the frequency of oral candidiasis in diabetic patients, we were interested in studying it in this study, which took place at the BATNA University Hospital.

Our main objective was to describe the epidemiological characteristics of BC in diabetics hospitalised in various departments (internal medicine, paediatrics, etc.).

And as secondary objectives :

- To determine the risk factors for the occurrence of BC in diabetics.
- Describe the different Candida species isolated.
- Establish a strategy for the proper management and prophylaxis of BC.

REVIEW OF LITTERATURE

1. ANATOMICAL OVERVIEW OF THE MOUTH

The mouth is the initial part of the digestive system, responsible for swallowing, mastication, gustation, insalivation and deglutition of food with the help of the activity of associated organs (teeth, tongue, salivary glands), and is also involved in communication, phonation and facial expression [6].

The mouth is also known as the oral cavity and is limited :
Forward: through the upper and lower lips.
Above: by the hard and soft palates that separate them from the nasal cavities. Below: by the floor of the mouth on which the tongue rests.
On the sides: through both cheeks
The oral cleft is the anterior opening of the oral cavity, communicating posteriorly with the oropharynx [6,7]. (Figure 1)

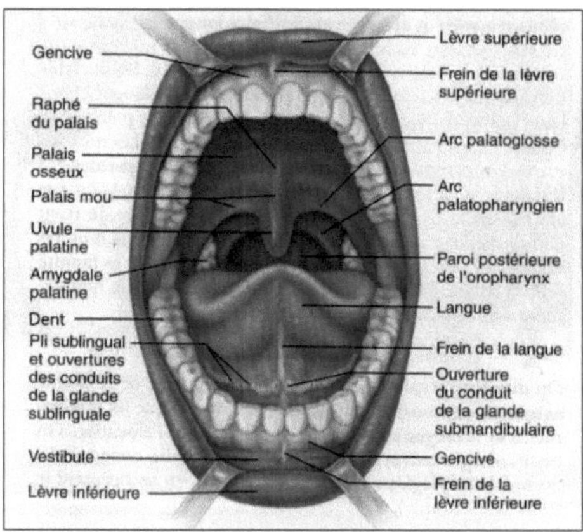

Figure 1: Anterior view of the oral cavity [6].

1.1 The lips

The lips are mobile muscular-membranous folds that delimit the oral cleft. They formed by the orbicularis muscle of the mouth, covered on the outside by the skin and on the inside by the glandular mucosa [7].

1.2 The cheeks

The cheeks form the lateral walls of the oral cavity, made up inside to outside by the buccal mucosa, the buccinator muscle and the skin [7].

1.3 The palace

It forms the roof of the mouth and has two parts:

- The anterior hard palate: separates the oral and nasal cavities. It is formed by a bony lamina covered on both the upper and lower sides by a mucous membrane and a rigid surface against which the tongue can push food away during chewing [7].

- The posterior soft palate: a mobile fold that separates the oropharynx from the

The is involved swallowing and sound modulation [6,7].

1.4 The language

The tongue is located on the floor of the mouth and consists of a fixed part, the root, and a free part, the body. The two parts are separated by the terminal sulcus [6].

The tongue is an organ of taste involved in chewing, swallowing and phonation [6].

1.5 Salivary glands

The salivary glands secrete saliva, which helps to protect the oral mucosa, chew and digest [6].

It includes the minor salivary glands and the major salivary glands (the parotid, submandibular and sublingual glands) [6].

1.6 The teeth

Teeth are implanted through the gums into the alveoli on the edges of the mandible and maxilla, which are hard organs designed for chewing food [6].

1.7 The oral mucosa

The oral mucosa is a richly vascularised and innervated membrane that lines the inner wall of the lips and the oral cavity. It covers the muscular and bony structures of the oral cavity [8,9].

It has a number of functions, the most important of which is to protect deep tissues. that it covers against compression and abrasion when eating [9].
In the event of injury, it acts as a protective barrier against the various micro-organisms by reproducing antimicrobial peptides called defensins [6].

The oral mucosa is made up a stratified squamous epithelium and a connective tissue called the chorion or lamina propria with a basement membrane separating the two [10].

Three types of mucosa are found in the oral cavity:

1.7.1 The masticatory mucosa

The mucosa is keratinised on the surface and lines the gum and hard palate. It is involved in the mechanical compression of food and has long epithelial ridges that invaginate deeply into the connective tissue [10].

1.7.2 The mucous membrane

The mucosa is non-keratinised on the surface and lines the mucosal surface of the lips, cheeks, floor, ventral surface the tongue and soft palate. It has epithelial ridges that are weakly anchored in the connective tissue [10].

The absence of keratinisation makes the mucosa thinner and therefore more fragile and more at risk. to develop precancerous lesions [10].

1.7.3 The mucous membrane of the dorsal surface of the tongue

This is a keratinised mucosa characterised by the presence of numerous papillae involved in the taste function (filiform papilla, fungiform papilla, caliciform papilla, taste buds, foliated papillae) [10].

2. DESCRIPTION AND MORPHOLOGY OF CANDIDA

2.1 Definition

The genus Candida was created at the IXth International Botanical Congress held in Canada in 1959, replacing the term Monilia, which had been used until then [11].

Candida is the abbreviated name used to describe a class of fungi that includes more than 150 species of yeast. In healthy people Candida exists harmlessly in mucous membranes (saprophyte) such as the gastrointestinal tract, mouth, urogenital tract, skin, etc. It is known as the "beneficial flora" and plays a useful role in the body. It is known as the "beneficial flora" and plays a useful role in the body [12].

Around 80% of infections are caused by Candida albicans, although infections due to non-albicans species such as: (Candida glabrata, Candida tropicalis, Candida parapsilosis, Candida krusei, Candida dubliniensis) are increasingly common [13].

Candidiasis may be superficial (e.g. oral, vaginal, mucocutaneous) or deep (e.g. myocarditis, pyelonephritis, meningitis, septicaemia, etc.) [13].

The relationship between Candida spp and candidiasis takes into account two important factors: Factors related to the microbe and factors related to host. An imbalance between these factors is associated with the pathogenicity of Candida spp [13].

2.2 Morphology

They are unicellular, yeast-like micromycetes characterised by a vegetative structure (the thallus) composed of spores [14,15].

The yeast or blastospore form is round or oval, varying in size from 2 to 4 µm in diameter, and generally reproduces asexually by budding [14,15].

Two filamentous forms can be found:

- A true mycelium: this is the continuous growth of the bud which gives rise to an elongated tubular structure, partitions appear secondarily to separate the articles, and it branches progressively giving an arborescent appearance [14,15].

- A pseudomycelium: this consists of a succession of elongated buds that remain attached to the mother cell and the preceding buds, resulting in a filamentous structure. Between each bud there is a constriction zone in which the blastospores develop and branch out, giving a bushy appearance [14,15].

Filamentation is favoured by a temperature above 37°C, an alkaline pH high concentrations of CO2, and is also favoured by a lack of nitrogen and carbon in the presence of N-acetylglucosamine [16].

With the exception of C.glabrata, Candida yeasts can produce filaments [15].

A particular feature of C.albicans and C.dubliniensis is that they also produce chlamydospores when environmental conditions are unfavourable. This feature is used for identification purposes [15]. (Figure 2).

The wall plays an important role in maintaining the integrity of the yeast, protecting it from environmental stresses such as osmotic changes, dehydration, temperature changes and also from the host's immune defences, and is responsible for the adhesion of the yeast to the host cell [15,16].

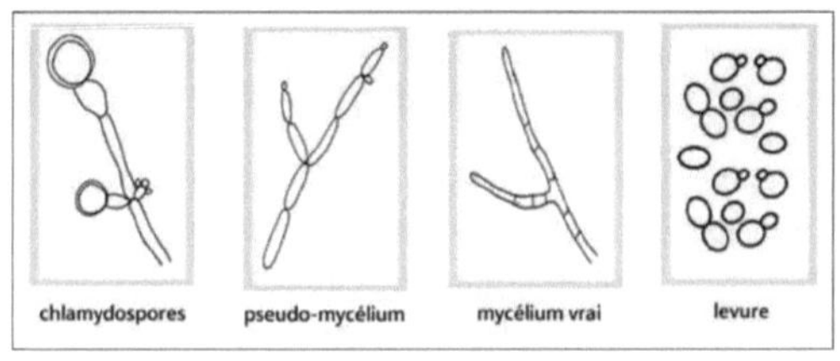

Figure 2: Different morphologies of the thallus [17].

2.3 Classification

The Candida genus is part of the Ascomycetes phylum, the Saccharomycetes class, the Saccharomycetales order and the mitosporic Saccharomycetales group. This classification is based on phenotypic characteristics and nucleotide sequence comparisons [18]. (Figure 3)

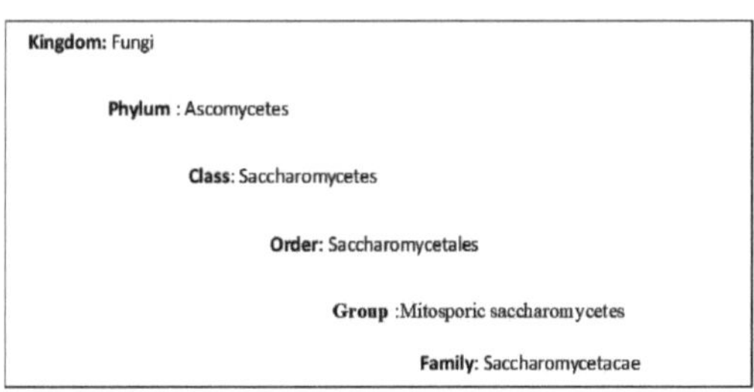

Figure 3: Position of the genus Candida in the current classification [18].

Candida species associated human infection :

Table 1: Candida species associated human infection [19].

Candida albicans	Candida dubliniensis
Candida parapsilosis	Candida tropicalis
Candida glabrata	Candida kefyr (pseudotropicalis)
Candida lusitaniae	Candida krusei
Candida guilliermondii	Candida utilis
Candida lipolytica	Candida famata
Candida haemulonii	Candida rugosa

3. PATHOPHYSIOLOGY OF ORAL CANDIDIASIS

Yeasts of the genus Candida are commensals of the natural cavities of man. In normal subjects, specific or non-specific defence elements and the ecology of the flora of the digestive tract, oropharyngeal sphere and vagina enable this commensal state to be maintained. In the normal host, Candida colonisation of the mucous membranes is not qualitatively and/or quantitatively significant enough to cause candidiasis [18].

The maintenance of this commensal state is part of a scenario in which the two players (the host and Candida), depending on their state (immunocompetent or immunocompromised patient, adaptive capacities of the yeasts expressing or not pathogenicity or virulence factors), develop their own strategy to counter the offensives of one or escape the defences of the other. The disruption of the balance governing this commensal state in favour of Candida, following the appearance of favouring factors in host, would result its becoming an opportunistic pathogen with the development of superficial or deep candidiasis [18].

Given the high prevalence of Candida as a harmless commensal in humans, it is not surprising that no primary virulence factors have been identified for this organism. However, a number of putative virulence factors have been proposed which, in the event of host debilitation, contribute to tissue damage and persistence of the micro-organism in the host [20].

These include :

3.1 The formation of biofilm

Biofilms are communities of micro-organisms embedded in an extracellular matrix, which confer significant resistance to antifungal treatments and enhance host immune responses. These communities can form on biotic surfaces (e.g. oral mucosa) or abiotic surfaces (e.g. catheters) [3].

The development of Candida spp biofilm can be explained in four chronological stages:

Adhesion: initial phase in which suspended yeast and planktonic cells adhere to the surface (1-3 h).Intermediate phase: biofilm development (11-14 h).

Maturation phase: the polymer matrix (PEM) completely penetrates all the layers of cells adhering to the surface in a three-dimensional structure (20-48 h).

Dispersion: the most superficial cells leave the biofilm and colonise the areas surrounding the surface (after 24 h).

Thus, a mature biofilm is made up a dense network of cells in the form of yeasts, hyphae or pseudohyphae (or not, depending on the Candida species) involved in PEM and water channels between the cells. The final architecture of the biofilm is variable and depends in part on the Candida spp involved, the growth conditions and the substrate on which it forms [3]. (Figure 4)

It is thought that high levels of glucose serve as the source of carbohydrate energy required by Candida spp for biofilm formation and are probably necessary to produce the polysaccharide matrix, which is secreted by sessile cells, providing protection against environmental challenges. Biofilms are refractory to antifungal agents and more difficult to treat than those formed with planktonic cells. In addition, Candida spp isolated from DM patients have been shown to have a higher pathogenic potential for biofilm formation [3].

In addition, biofilms formed by isolates of C. albicans, C. parapsilosis, C. tropicalis and C. glabrata were associated with higher morbidity and mortality rates than isolates unable to form biofilms [20].

In addition, biofilms on an oral prosthesis, usually a denture, are a major predisposing factor for chronic oral candidiasis. Candida readily adhere to the polymethylacrylate materials of dentures, and also exploit microcracks and fissures in the materials to facilitate retention [20].

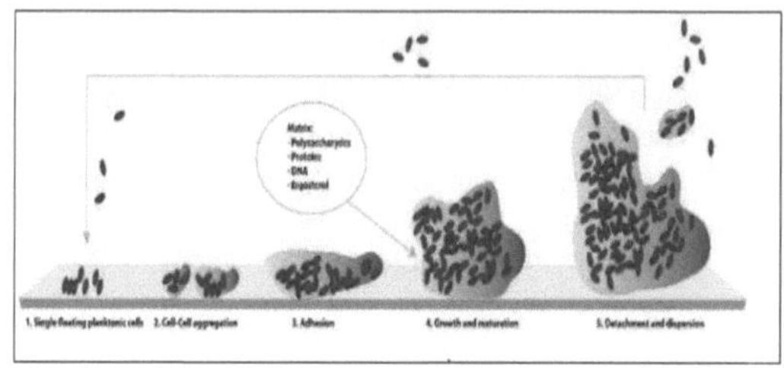

Figure 4: Development a Candida spp biofilm on a surface [3].

3.2 Hydrophobia

In Candida spp, adhesion is mediated by agglutinin-like (Als) proteins, which are linked by glycosylphosphatidylinositol to the β-1-6 glucans of the fungal cell wall. Als-dependent cell adhesion is linked to an increase in hydrophobicity of the cell surface (CSH). Candida spp CSH increases virulence by promoting adhesion to host tissues [3].

Hydrophobicity is a virulent factor that is gene-regulated and generally positively correlated biofilm metabolic activity, since hydrophobic interactions appear to be crucial in promoting tissue invasion by the mycelial phase of Candida spp [3].

It is assumed that Candida spp can grow under anaerobic conditions, under these conditions fermentation is the dominant pathway for ATP . The results of Sardi et al indicate that 51.97% of isolates from diabetic patients were highly hydrophobic under anaerobic conditions, compared with 21.90% in an aerobic atmosphere [3].

3.3 Enzymes hydrolytic

Several studies have established an association between the activity of hydrolytic enzymes and an increase in the pathogenic capacity of Candida spp. It has been shown that, due to a higher concentration of glucose in the blood in diabetics, Candida spp isolates have a significantly higher haemolytic and esterase enzymatic activity, which may contribute to increased enzymatic activity. The same authors also hypothesised that these species are more pathogenic under abnormal conditions such as diabetes [3].

The destruction of host tissues by Candida species can be facilitated by the release of hydrolytic enzymes into the local environment. Secreted aspartyl proteinases (SAPs), phospholipases (PLs), lipases and haemolysins are the enzymes most frequently implicated in the pathogenicity of Candida species [21].

SAPs facilitate invasion and colonisation of host tissues by disrupting host mucosal membranes and degrading important immunological and structural defence proteins [21].

Secreted SAPs capable of degrading many substrates that constitute host proteins in the oral cavity have also been studied. These enzymes are thought to help Candida spp acquire the nitrogen essential for growth, attach to and penetrate the oral mucosa, or both. They can also cause increased vascular permeability, leading to inflammatory reactions and clinical symptoms [3].

In addition to SAPs, enzymes classified as phospholipases are often thought to be involved in Candida pathogenicity. Phospholipases are enzymes that hydrolyse phospholipids into fatty acids. Production of all classes of phospholipases has been described for Candida species and it is suggested that they contribute to damage of the host cell membrane, which may also expose receptors to facilitate adhesion [21].

Similarly, PL targets membrane phospholipids and digests these components, initiating cell lysis and facilitating the penetration of infecting fungi. This enzyme induces the accumulation of inflammatory cells and plasma proteins, releasing several inflammatory mediators in vivo [3].

Haemolysins are substances that lyse red blood cells, their production by Candida is considered an important attribute in promoting survival within host through an increased ability to sequester iron. Luo et al α and β haemolysis by clinical isolates of C. albicans, C. dubliniensis, C. kefyr, C. krusei, C. zeylanoides, C. glabrata, C. tropicalis and C. lusitaniae [20].

Haemolysin production is positively correlated with glucose concentration and this could be a predictive factor for candidiasis in poorly controlled diabetics where blood and salivary glucose levels are higher [20].

3.4 Variability genomic

Genomic variability is very common in Candida spp and is one of the factors that give this microbial group diversity in terms of increased virulence, adaptation to new environments or resistance to antifungal drugs. The presence of hyper-variable sub-populations in natural populations enables Candida spp to adapt rapidly to periods of stress. Genome rearrangements by recombination, loss heterozygosity, copy number variations, the presence of short tandem repeats or transposable elements, chromosomal inversions or mutations such as deletions, insertions or single-nucleotide polymorphisms are ways in which Candida species achieve their evolutionary history. In pathogenic Candida spp, almost all CTG codons are translated to serine instead of leucine, thus masking β-glucan and interfering with host recognition. Genomic plasticity differs between Candida species. It is clear that C. albicans has both the most complex genome (including virulence genes such as SAP) and the most ways of ensuring its genomic diversity, making the microorganism-host interaction unpredictable, depending on the balance between virulence factors and the host immune response [13].

3.5 Morphological plasticity of Candida spp

Candida spp can undergo a reversible morphological transition to better penetrate host epithelial barrier. Yeast cells can take different forms: unicellular budding yeast cells or filamentous forms such as hyphae or pseudohyphae, each playing a distinct role in the invasion process of the infection. Although the formation of hyphae is considered to be a virulence factor, the filamentation process only begins after adhesion to the host surface. Morphogenesis is a virulence factor for two main reasons: hyphal formation facilitates the invasion process and helps C. albicans to defend itself against the immune system. Hyphae pierce host cells and, because they are larger than yeast cells, are more difficult for the immune system to kill. In addition, C. albicans can kill macrophages. The killing process involves the formation of hyphae, followed by elongation, stretching and puncturing of the macrophage cell membrane [13].

4. RISK FACTORS FOR ORAL CANDIDIASIS

Candida can colonise the oral cavity without causing any lesions. This colonisation occurs when there is an imbalance between the virulence factors of the fungus and the host's defences. The combination of various intrinsic and extrinsic factors predisposes to the transition from the saprophytic to the pathogenic state and the risk of disease development.

4.1 Intrinsic factors

4.1.1 Immune deficiencies

- **Physiological immunosuppression**

The extreme ages of life (premature babies, newborns and the elderly) are the risk groups most exposed to oral candidiasis [22].

In newborns, the immaturity of their immune system combined with the still incomplete development of their microbial flora favours this infection and it can be transmitted in different ways, in most cases acquired intrapartum through contact with contaminated vaginal mucosa, or during breastfeeding via the mother's breast or hands, inadequately sterilised feeding bottles or food. For this reason, the incidence of oral candidiasis is 1 to 37% higher in bottle-fed newborns than in breast-fed babies [23].

- **Congenital immunodepression**

Primary immune deficiency is a group of diseases characterised by the diversity of genetic disorders affecting the molecules responsible for the immune response, resulting in a deficiency in the means of defence, generally CD4 lymphocytes, and consequently increased susceptibility to fungal infections [22].

- **Acquired immunodepression**

AIDS, thymic disorders, haematological malignancies and sarcoidosis increase the susceptibility of oral candidiasis [24].Oral candidiasis is the most common opportunistic infection in HIV infection [24].

According to the CDC "Centres of disease control" classification in Atlanta, revised in 1993, it is considered to be a pathology revealing AIDS, classified in category B, and it is estimated that more than 90% of HIV-infected patients develop this infection during the progression of their disease [24,25].

4.1.2 Terrain endocrine

The various Candida species are more frequently isolated from the oral cavity of diabetic patients than non-diabetic patients. Among the factors that predispose diabetic patients to oral candidiasis are the high levels of salivary glucose, which allow glycosylation of proteins on the surface of host epithelial cells during glycaemic peaks. This increase in glycosylated residues increases the number of receptors for Candida and alters the chemotactic activity of neutrophils [26,27].
Candida-associated lesions including prosthetic stomatitis, median rhomboid glossitis and angular cheilitis have been reported to be more common in patients with diabetes [27].
Pregnancy, Cushing's syndrome, hypoparathyroidism, thyroid insufficiency

and adrenal glands are among the risk factors for candidiasis [28,29].

4.1.3 Local factors

- **Hyposialia (xerostomia)**

Saliva plays a major role in maintaining the health of the oral cavity. Insufficient saliva secretion or changes in its composition encourage the development of oral candidiasis [30].

Studies have shown that in diabetic patients, hyperglycaemia has an effect on the reduction in salivary flow, which can lead to a number of oral and dental problems:

• Acidification of the oral environment due to the reduction in pH encourages yeast proliferation.

• Decrease in the action of several antimicrobial factors which will create a environment conducive to the proliferation of pathogenic microorganisms [31].
These changes generally delay healing and increase susceptibility to infection, cheilitis, dry mucous membranes with fissures, chapped lips and an increase in the prevalence of dental caries [32].The lack oral hygiene assessed on brushing combined with the wearing of a removable dental prosthesis thus encourages the development oral candidiasis [30].

4.1.4 Nutritional deficiencies

Nutritional deficiencies can lead to a reduction in host defence and loss of epithelial integrity, which can facilitate fungal invasion. It is well known that a diet rich in carbohydrates can favour oral candidiasis. Iron deficiency helps to reduce cellular immunity by reducing the bactericidal activity of PNNs, as well as leading to an inadequate humoral immunity response and epithelial abnormalities in anaemic subjects. Vitamin B12 and folic acid deficiency cause leukocyte and platelet abnormalities, as well as particularly marked changes in the oral epithelium due to their rapid renewal [22,27].

4.1.5 Malignant diseases

Cancers and bone marrow aplasias and their treatment lead to significant immunosuppression, and also cause a loss of integrity of the oral mucosa and destruction of other structures such as the salivary glands, taste buds and periodontium. This leads to oral ulcerations and hyposialia associated with an imbalance in the oral flora [29].

4.2 Extrinsic factors

4.2.1 The medicines

Broad-spectrum antibiotics (ATBs) alter the saprophytic oral flora, which will promote yeast proliferation, and this risk increases with the length of use [33].
Immunosuppressive drugs predispose to oral candidiasis by altering the oral flora, disturbing the mucosal surface and changing the character of saliva [33].

Radiotherapy and antitumour chemotherapy thus lead to a reduction in immunity favourable to the development of Candida [30].
In addition, anticholinergic drugs, particularly psychotropic drugs (antidepressants and neuroleptics), may be responsible for hyposialia and increase the risk of oral candidiasis [30].

4.2.2 Chronic alcoholism and smoking

Excessive consumption damages the lining of the oesophagus, which can lead to Candida colonisation [34].
Smoking causes changes in the pigmentation of teeth, alters the sense of smell and taste, and slows down and disrupts wound healing during dental surgery, such as extractions. It is also

considered to be a significant risk indicator for increased caries activity, and is linked increased susceptibility to oral candidiasis [34].

5. CLINICAL ASPECTS OF ORAL CANDIDIASIS

5.1 Acute pseudomembranous candidiasis

Also known as acute thrush, this is the most common form and generally appears as a whitish or yellowish-white coating reminiscent of curdled milk that covers the oral mucosa, labial surface, palate, tongue, periodontium and oropharynx and is easily detached, revealing an erosive red mucosa. Patients may complain of a metallic taste sensation and dryness [15,35].

It occurs in people of extreme age, during diabetes and in HIV patients, and also affects patients taking inhaled corticosteroids, antibiotics, psychotropic drugs or chemotherapy [15,35].

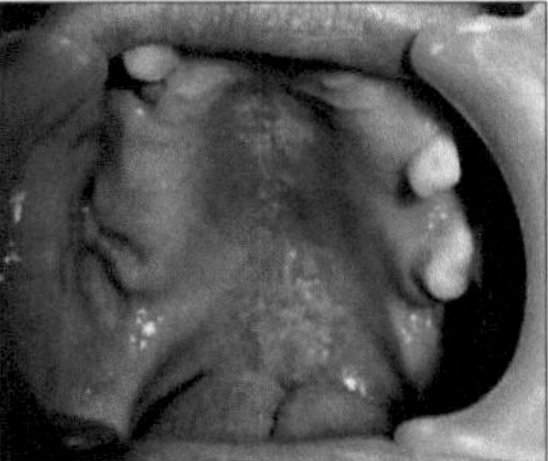

Figure 5: Pseudomembranous candidiasis in an asthmatic patient taking inhaled corticosteroids [27].

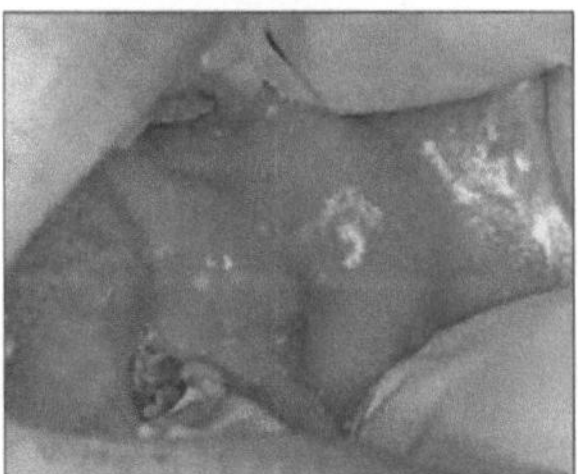

Figure 6: Pseudomembranous candidiasis of the left cheek [36].

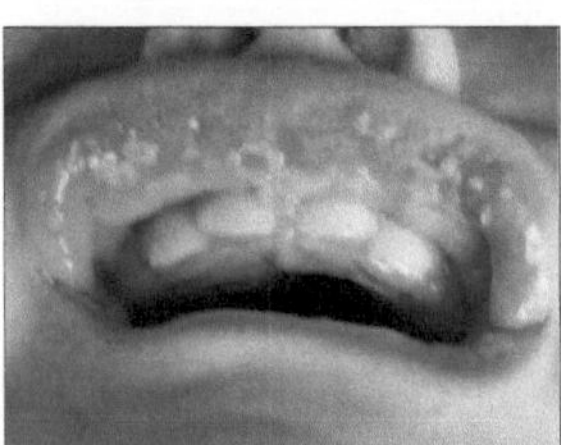

Figure 7: Pseudomembranous candidiasis in infants [36].

5.2 Acute atrophic erythematous candidiasis

This type of candidiasis occurs in the context broad-spectrum antibiotic therapy, following a reduction in the levels of bacterial flora, which facilitates the proliferation of Candida, or when aerosol corticosteroids are taken. It may precede or be the consequence of acute pseudomembranous candidiasis, the oral mucosa is inflammatory red with no whitish plaque, and the tongue is vermilion and depilated. It is a painful form of burn [15,37].

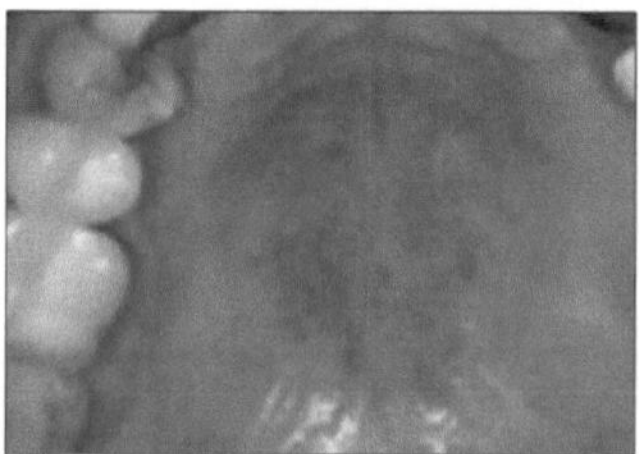

Figure 8.Erythematous atrophic candidiasis in an elderly subject [30].

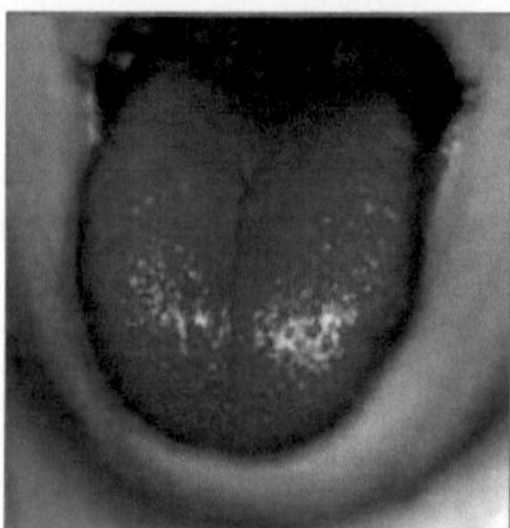

Figure 9.Erythematous candidiasis with perlchea [38].

5.3 Chronic atrophic erythematous candidiasis

Known as prosthetic stomatitis, it generally occurs in people who wear dentures day and night. Prosthetic stomatitis is seen in up to 75% of denture wearers [37]. Other factors predispose the subject to prosthetic stomatitis: poor oral hygiene, thumb-sucking habit and dental trauma due to unsuitable prostheses [37]. Clinically, it is characterised by chronic erythema of the tissues covered by the dental prosthesis. Pain is slight or absent, and oral lesions are associated with angular cheilitis [15,33].

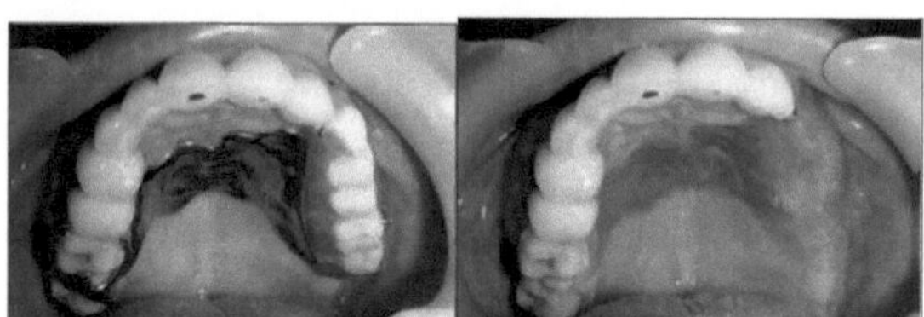

Figure 10.Prosthetic stomatitis showing localised erythema of the tissues covered by the denture [27].

5.4 Chronic pseudomembranous candidiasis

This is an untreated acute case of thrush which has developed into a chronic condition. The predisposing factors are the same as for the acute form [15].
In this condition, whitish coatings adhere to an erythematous mucosa [15].

5.5 Chronic hyperplastic candidiasis

Also known as pseudotumour candidiasis, it is characterised by hard-to-remove plaques on the inner surface of the cheeks and the sides of the tongue. There is a risk of malignant transformation of this type lesion [16,35].

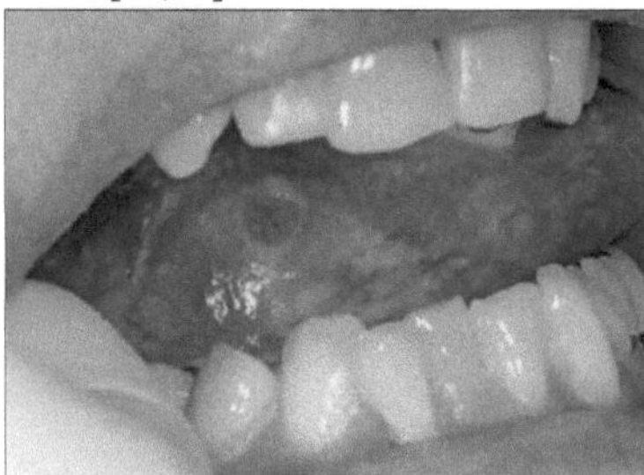

Figure 11.Hyperplastic candidiasis with traumatic ulcer changes due to friction[36].

5.6 Angular cheilitis or perlèche

It presents as cracks and crusts in the labial commissures. There are several aetiologies implicating the occurrence of this form: the wearing of unsuitable dental prostheses, xerostomia, licking, bruxism and vitamin B deficiency [15]. Angular cheilitis is most often an opportunistic fungal and/or bacterial infection [15].

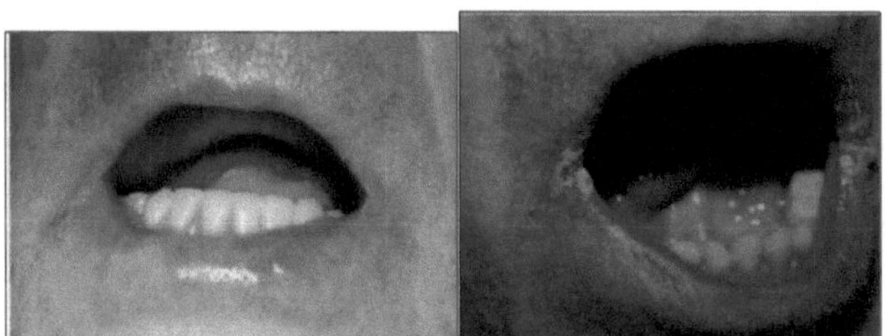

Figure 12.angular cheilitis or perlecheitis in an elderly subject [30,37].

5.7 Chronic candidiasis at

This form is seen in non-insulin-dependent diabetic patients and smokers [15]. There are two aspects:

5.7.1 Median glossitis rhombic

Also known as central papillary atrophy, this is a condition that affects the organ system. In this case, the organ affected is the tongue, and the patient complains of tingling or burning on contact with spicy or acidic foods [15].

It is a medio-lingual depapillated rhomboid [15].

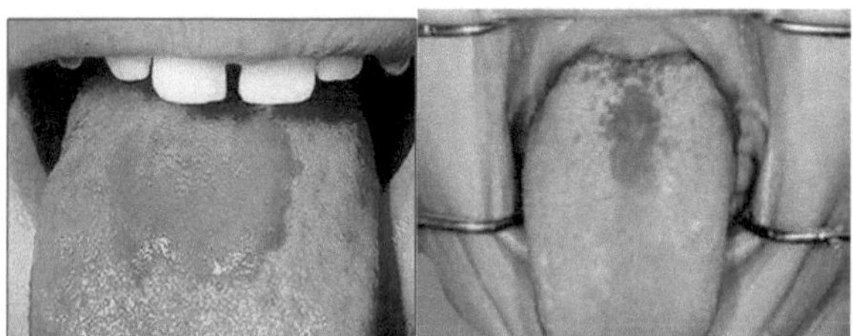

Figure 13: Median rhombic glossitis [36,38].

5.7.2 Median ouranite posterior

It is characterised by an erythematous area surrounded a red patch. corresponding to the inflammatory ostia of the salivary glands [15].

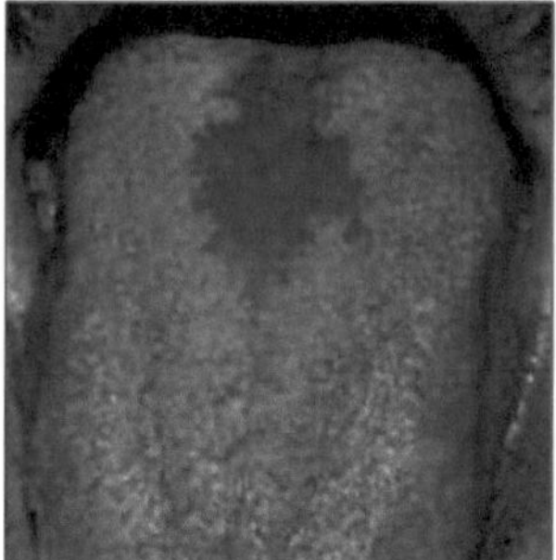

Figure 14.Erythematous form associated with median ouranitis in an HIV+ patient [39].

5.8 White tongue saburrale

This form is characterised by a whitish coating that covers the tongue, is frequently observed in cases of digestive disorders and may be of infectious origin, caused by a fungus of the Candida genus [15].

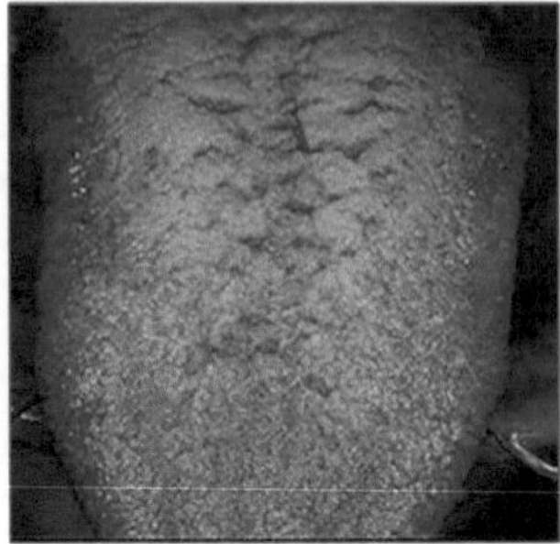

Figure 15.Sabral white tongue [40].

5.9 Black tongue

This is a fairly common form, characterised by elongation and hypertrophy of the ends of the papillae, leading to the formation of villi which turn black. These papillae are agglomerated by a mucopolysaccharide coating derived from saliva. The black colour is thought to be due to oxidation and the chromogenic nature of certain bacteria [15]. Poor oral hygiene, digestive pathologies, alcohol consumption or smoking and the oxidative effect of certain ATBs have been suggested as contributing to the development of this condition [15].

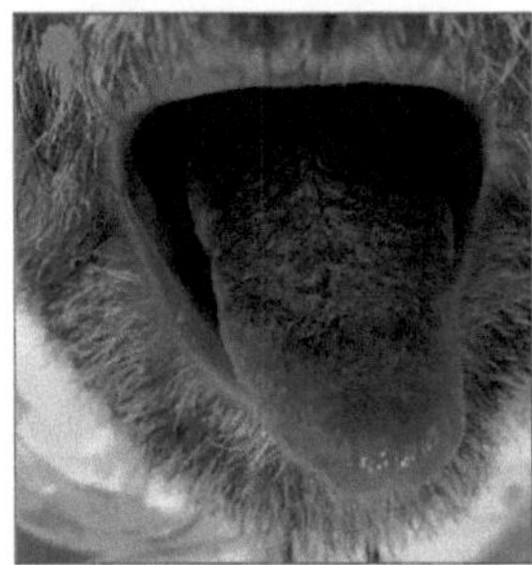

Figure 16: Black tongue in an elderly patient [41].

6. DIAGNOSIS OF ORAL CANDIIDOSIS

Diagnosis of oral candidiasis is essentially clinical, based on recognition of the lesions, and can be confirmed by microscopic identification of Candida in oral swabs and/or isolation in culture [42].

The detection of Candida in the oral cavity is not indicative of infection, as it is a common commensal micro-organism in this area. A definitive diagnosis of candidiasis requires confirmation tissue invasion by Candida. This underlines the importance of clinical diagnosis of the disease [42].

6.1 Diagnosis clinical

The history, followed a thorough examination of the mouth, soft palate and hard palate, as well as the buccal mucosa in people wearing dentures after they have been removed, is generally a good starting point. The correct diagnosis is usually made on the basis of the finding of the characteristic lesion, exclusion of other possibilities and the response to antifungal treatment [33].

A mycological study is generally necessary when there are diagnostic doubts, when there is resistance to antifungal drugs or when the dose of antifungal drug needs to be adjusted, such as in immunocompromised patients. Mycological techniques are also used when it is necessary to control the disease in order to prevent infection spreading further, and when the Candida species needs to be identified in order to establish the most effective treatment. Biopsies are always necessary in hyperplastic candidiasis to rule out epithelial dysplasia [42].

Yeasts can be identified on the basis of four different criteria: morphological and biochemical (for the diagnosis of oral candidiasis), or immunological and genetic (for the diagnosis of invasive candidiasis or the differentiation of species such as C. albicans and C. dubliniensis) [42].

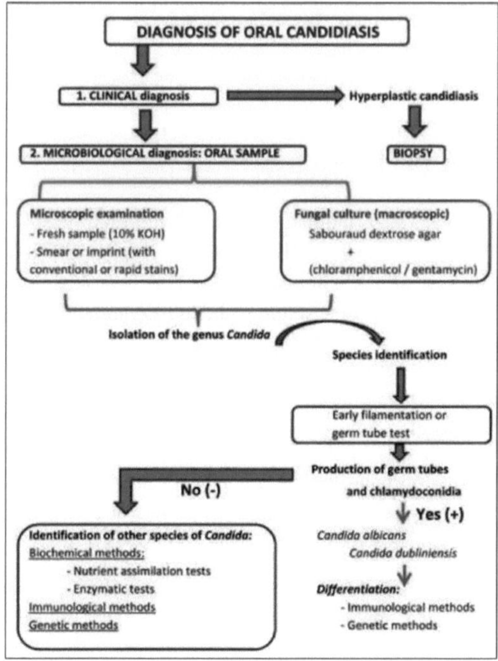

Figure 17.Diagnosis of oral candidiasis [42].

6.2 Diagnosis microbiology

6.2.1 Examination microscopic

Microscopic examination can be carried out with fresh samples, using 10% potassium hydroxide (KOH), which dissolves the epithelial cells and leaves Candida intact, or 15-30% sodium hydroxide (NaOH). It is also possible prepare smears or impressions of lesion samples, followed by conventional Giemsa or PAS staining, or rapid techniques such as Gram staining. In the case of hyperplastic candidiasis, a biopsy of the lesions is usually obtained and stained with haematoxylin-eosin (showing yeast and fungi). purple Candida pseudomycelia), PAS or Gomori-Grocott Methenamine Silver [42].

6.2.2 Mycological culture

Macroscopic observation is carried out on culture plates. The culture medium used is Sabouraud dextrose agar, which allows selective fungal growth. Chloramphenicol 0.05 g/l or Gentamycin 0.5 g/l is usually added to this medium to inhibit bacterial growth. Cycloheximide 0.05 g can also be added, as it prevents the proliferation of other accompanying fungi. After incubation (24-48 hours), smooth, shiny, whitish colonies are observed [42].

6.2.3 Identification of species

6.2.3.1 The filamentation test (blastèse test)

Using cultures, we can isolate the Candida genus and identify the species. For the identification of C. albicans, we use the early filamentation test or the germ tube test. Cornstarch agar, oxgall-preado-caffeic acid, diluted milk and various sera, such as horse serum, can be used for such tests. Horse serum is the most commonly used option, with incubation at 37°C for 2-3 hours. After the incubation period, we can observe the characteristic germ tubes of C. albicans [42].

6.2.3.2 The chlamydosporulation test

On PCB (potato, carrot, marble) and RAT (rice, agar, tween 80) media, C. albicans produces chlamydospores at the end of pseudomycelium in 24 to 48 h at 25-28°C, while C. dubliniensis produces chlamydospores in greater numbers, arranged in pairs or triplets [15].

The identification of germ tubes and chlamydoconidia is indicative of an infection produced by C. albicans and/or C. dubliniensis, whereas their absence is indicative of a probable infection due to non-C. albicans species [42].

6.2.3.3 Biochemical methods

other Candida species need to be evaluated, we can biochemical methods, including enzymatic techniques, methods and mixed techniques that combine enzymatic and nutrient assimilation tests. Enzymatic techniques (chromogenic media, commercial media for rapid identification of C. albicans and commercial methods for rapid identification of C. glabrata) detect the activity of certain yeast enzymes by the specific hydrolysis of a chromogenic substrate in the presence of an enzymatic indicator. Numerous enzymatic techniques are commercially available (CHROMagar Candida®, Candida® ID, etc.). However, the most frequently used system is CHROMagar Candida®, where C. albicans grows forming smooth green colonies, C. tropicalis forms smooth blue colonies and C. krusei forms rough pink colonies. Another widely used chromogenic method is Candida ID®, where C. albicans grows to form smooth blue colonies, C. tropicalis and C. guillermondii generate pink colonies, and the rest of species appear as white colonies. In terms of the sensitivity and specificity of chromogenic methods, CHROMagar Candida® and Candida ID® are simple, easy to use, accessible and offer good sensitivity and specificity, as they allow presumptive identification of most Candida species [42].

Among the range of biochemical techniques, nutrient uptake tests assess the fungal ability to use different sugars as a single carbon source. Media containing all the essential elements for growth, with the exception of one carbon source, are used. A certain sugar is then added to the medium, and the ability of the fungus to assimilate this sugar is demonstrated by its growth in the culture medium. This technique produces what is known as an auxanogram. The auxanogram can be obtained using conventional techniques, commercial micromethods or automated systems. Numerous techniques are currently available to facilitate the use of these tests, making them faster but also more expensive. Nutrient assimilation tests include Auxacolor®, Uni- Yeast-Tek®, API 20 C AUX®... Finally, among biochemical methods, a number of commercial techniques combine enzymatic tests and nutrient assimilation techniques, such as Rapid Yeast Plus System® and Fongiscreen 4H® [42].

6.2.3.4 immunological methods

C. dubliniensis produces germ tubes and chlamydospores in the same way as C. albicans. In order distinguish between them, we therefore need to apply immunological and genetic criteria. Such criteria are also used to diagnose invasive candidiasis. Immunological criteria are used in patients with complicated clinical conditions (such as the immunocompromised), when it is difficult to obtain deep samples or when there are long waiting intervals between cultures. Immunological techniques include methods based on mannan/anti-mannan detection (Platelia™ Candida Ab/Ac/Ak), antimycelial antibody detection (Candida albicans IFA IgG), other antibody detection (Candida Detect™) and (1-3) β-D-glucan detection (Fungitec G, Wako, B-Gstar). Immunological procedures also include latex particle agglutination , based on the use of specific monoclonal antibodies (Bichro-latex albicans®, Krusei-color®, Bichro-Dubli®) [42].

6.2.3.5 Genetic methods

Genetic techniques offer high sensitivity and specificity, and allow identification of the pathogen without the need for cultures. In addition, samples from patients receiving antifungal treatment can be used; however, these techniques are more expensive and are not available in most hospitals. Molecular diagnosis is based on nucleic acid hybridisation and amplification techniques. The aim of genetic systems is to identify yeasts directly in clinical samples without the need to extract nucleic acids, thereby eliminating culture time and reducing costs. Bosco-Borgeat et al. and Liguori et al, have proposed multiplex polymerase chain reaction (PCR) assays, as they meet the above objective; however, although these assays are valid, they remain expensive [42].

7. TREATMENT OF ORAL CANDIDIASIS

The management of oral candidiasis is based on four principles:

1- Early and accurate diagnosis of the infection.

2- Correct predisposing factors or underlying diseases.

3- Assess the clinical aspect of oral Candida candidiasis.

4- Appropriate use of antifungal agents, assessing the efficacy/toxicity ratio on a case-by-case basis.

When choosing between certain treatments, it is important to take into account the species of Candida, its clinical form and whether it should be combined with a topical treatment or a more complex systemic treatment, always evaluating the efficacy/toxicity ratio [43].

The aims of treatment are to identify and eliminate possible contributing factors, prevent systemic spread and eliminate any associated discomfort. Pharmacological treatment must be tailored to each patient, depending on their current state of health, the clinical presentation and the severity of the infection [43].

Before initiating treatment, it is first necessary to eliminate the factors that can be identified as contributing to the disease, in order to improve the therapeutic outcome and reduce the likelihood of recurrence of candidiasis:

- Diabetes management.
- Restore good oral hygiene by using mouthwashes with anti-Candida activity, in particular triclosan and chlorhexidine gluconate, and by using essential oils (EOs), which contain natural plant extracts such as :

Allium cepa 'onion', Allium sativum 'garlic', Allium schoenoprasum 'chives', Allium tuberosum 'Chinese chives'. Several pharmacological activities have been attributed to these species, including anti-diabetic, hepatoprotective, anti-parasitic and antibacterial activity, and above all antifungal activity against isolates of C. parapsilosis and inhibitory effects on biofilm formation [44].

Cinnamomum cassia 'Chinese cinnamon' is thought to be active against C. albicans and C. tropicalis,

C. glabrata and C. krusei, it is effective in reducing the number of pseudohyphae C. albicans cultures, which is considered an important virulence factor [44].

Tests have also demonstrated the anti-proliferative activity C cassia EO against Candida [44].

Some studies have reported that Cinnamomum zeylanicum 'Ceylon cinnamon' EO has antifungal activity against Candida Spp, most probably by disrupting the yeast cell wall [44,45].

Coriandrum sativum 'coriander' is widely used as a cholesterol-lowering agent, digestive stimulant, anti-hypertensive, antibacterial and antioxidant [44,45].

Coriander EO has also been shown to have a powerful antifungal effect against Candida, acting in a similar way to Nystatin and Amphotericin B [44,45].

Citral, an agent naturally present in many citric fruits, has been shown to have fungicidal activity against Candida [44].

Thymol, an aromatic compound found in thyme, has been reported to have a powerful antifungal effect against Candida strains by acting on the fungal cell membrane and producing a synergistic effect when used with Nystatin to inhibit the growth of these strains [44].

Sabzghabaee et al, evaluated the clinical efficacy of a gel containing Pelargonium graveolens EO for the treatment of prosthetic stomatitis. Another clinical study, conducted by Amanlou et al, showed that Zataria multiflora EO is also effective in treating prosthetic stomatitis. Denture wearers applied a gel containing 0.1% Zataria multiflora EO four times a day for a fortnight. The presence of erythema on the surface of the participants' palates was considerably reduced, as was the number of yeast strains [44].

Curcumin exhibits antifungal activity through various mechanisms, such as targeting metabolic pathways, inducing apoptosis and increasing reactive oxygen species. These properties of curcumin are effective in designing drug formulations with fewer side effects and superior performance. Narayanan et al, evaluated inhibitory action of curcumin against C. albicans, C. parapsilosis, C. glabrata and C. dublieniensis, proving its potential as a therapeutic alternative to conventional antifungals [44,45].

- Denture fitting and the need to remove it at night and wash it properly by leaving it immersed a disinfectant solution will benefit the elimination of the layer of biofilm generated in the prosthetic surface.
- Stop smoking.
- Treatment : corticosteroids, immunosuppressants, antibiotics.

For patients using steroid inhalers, it is important to brush and rinse the roof of the mouth after each use. Refer the patient to the pharmacist to review the appropriate aerosol inhalation technique and consider the need for an alternative inhalation chamber and metered dose inhaler, if required [38,46].

Curative treatment

As far as pharmacological treatment of candidiasis is concerned, a distinction can be made between two procedures: topical medications, which are applied to the affected area and treat superficial infections, and systemic medications, which are prescribed when the infection is more widespread and has not been sufficiently treated with topical therapy [43].

Treatment of oral mycoses is initially local. It can be started in the form of compound mouthwashes (Éludril® 90 ml, Fungizone® 60 ml, 14bicarbonated water 500 ml), when the clinical examination is inconclusive or while waiting for the results of mycological sampling. This magistral preparation is very well tolerated and improves oral comfort, but it has the disadvantage of being unstable and should be kept cool (refrigerator). If the mycosis is clinically evident, antifungal treatment can be started immediately without waiting for the results of the swab [38].

In the case of early or slightly lesions

It is based on the first-line prescription a local antifungal agent:

Nystatin (Mycostatin) or Amphotericin B (Fungizone) orally or the application a Miconazole gel (Daktarin gel) for 3 to 4 times a day between meals for a period of 7 to 15 days, it is necessary for the product to remain in contact with the oral mucosa for 2 to 3 minutes [43].
Miconazole (Loramyc) 50 mg gingival tablet, 1cp/d in the morning for 7 days, can also be used [43].

In patients wearing , when rinsing with the topical antifungal, the dentures must be removed to ensure good contact between the drug and the affected mucosa [43].

In the event of relapses or more lesions

In immunocompromised patients or after repeated failures of local treatments, systemic antifungal agents are prescribed [43].
Fluconazole (Triflucan) is well tolerated and is recommended as a first-line treatment, unless the isolated species is C. krusei or C. glabrata. The daily dose is 50 to 100 mg, depending on the intensity of the lesions and the patient's condition, 1 tablet per day for 7 to 14 days [43].
Various studies have shown that it is a very effective drug against pseudomembranous candidiasis, as it adheres well to the surface of the oral mucosa and has a rapid symptomatic response [43].
Another alternative is to prescribe Itraconazole [43].

If this fails, Voriconazole, Posaconazole or

Capsofungine [43].

In forms

Systemic treatment with Fluconazole 100 mg/d/15 d is recommended. It is necessary to specify the Candida species involved and that these treatment regimens do not contribute to the emergence of resistant strains, particularly for C. krusei and C. glabrata [15].

8. PROPHYLAXIS OF ORAL CANDIDIASIS

As prevention is the most effective treatment, much more so than eradicating yeast with synthetic or natural antifungal agents, it is essential to address and modify predisposing factors. It is therefore essential to good personal hygiene [47].

Prevention is ensured by good hygiene practices and particular attention to the adaptation of dental prostheses to avoid the proliferation of Candida spp and to limit the adverse effects of traditional antifungal agents [45].

Progress has been made in the development of anti-Candida biomaterials, and by using polymeric, inorganic and natural products that are intrinsically fungistatic or fungicidal, several strategies can be developed to prevent the proliferation of Candida spp [45].

Functionalisation and/or incorporation of these products into denture base materials are all considered to be effective new treatment options for oral candidiasis [45].

The presence of Candida biofilms reduces the likelihood of the organisms being eliminated by host defence mechanisms and antifungal agents. Appropriate management of biofilms is therefore essential. There is no single approach that can be taken to specifically combat Candida biofilms, and various mechanical and chemical methods aimed at improving oral hygiene are generally adopted. Ideally, an anti-biofilm approach will prevent biofilm development in the first place, as well as being effective against established biofilms. Standard oral hygiene practices, including tooth brushing and the use of mouthwashes, are important [19].

Probiotics could be used regularly as a prophylactic or therapeutic means, without side effects, to reduce Candida. Probiotics are live micro-organisms that are administered in adequate quantities. The concept behind their use in the treatment of oral candidiasis would be to exert microbiological pressure in the local environment, either by competing for adhesion sites and nutrients, or by creating an environment that is not conducive to the growth of Candida. Probiotics also appear to have beneficial effects on immune modulation [19,48]. Probiotics also reduce the risk of hyposalivation and the sensation of dry mouth, and can therefore be considered beneficial for oral health in general [48].

It is no less important to avoid certain risk factors, such as diets high in sugar and low in vitamins and minerals, or the use of antibiotics. frequency of use of ATBs, duration, amplitude and quantities should be kept to a minimum [47].

Rinsing the mouth after using an inhaled steroid is useful in preventing oral candidiasis [49].

Glucose promotes yeast growth, and a diet rich in carbohydrates increases their adhesion to oral epithelial cells [49].

Limiting their consumption is useful in controlling Candida colonisation and oral infection [49].

Mechanical removal of Candida plaques or heavy biofilm from oral lesions can improve antifungal action and speed healing [49].

Underlying predisposing factors must be identified and treated simultaneously, and monitored regularly [49].

MATERIALS AND METHODS

1. Equipment

1.1 Framework of the study

The study took place at the Benflis Touhami University Hospital (CHU Batna), in the following departments:

1. Paediatrics department; paediatric inpatient unit and nursery.
2. Internal Medicine Department; male and female inpatient units.
3. Orthopaedics and Traumatology ; men's, women's and children's inpatient unit.
4. Cardiology department; inpatient unit for men and women.

Oral swabs are then processed in the parasitology and medical mycology department of Batna University Hospital.

1.2 Type of study

This is a prospective descriptive cross-sectional study, based on the observation of the oral condition, particularly the oral mucosa, and the evaluation of the frequency of oral candidiasis and the risk factors involved in the occurrence of this disease in hospitalised diabetic patients of different ages over a period of five (5) months from 01st November 2021 to 31 March 2022.

1.3 Population of the study

All diabetic patients treated at the Batna Hospital Centre who agreed to answer the questionnaire.

- **Inclusion :**

• Diabetic patients of different ages and sexes, previously diagnosed with this disease.
• Patients recently diagnosed with diabetes mellitus.
• Diabetic patients consenting to take part in our study.

- **Exclusion :**

• Diabetic patients followed at Batna University Hospital who did not agree to answer the questionnaires and/or undergo an oral-dental examination during our study period.

1.4 Collection of data

The data was collected from information sheets containing the following information general and specific information on oral candidiasis. For general information, we looked for the following for all patients: hospital ward, type and age of diabetes, sex, age, reason for and duration of hospitalisation, medical and surgical history, and treatment received. Information specific to oral candidiasis was sought on: hygiene and dietetic measures, tooth brushing, visits to the dentist and clinical signs in the oral cavity (see appendix 1).

1.5 Processing and analysis of data

We carried out a manual tabulation to classify the data according to target. The data collected was entered and analysed using Excel 2016 software.

1.6 Laboratory equipment

1.6.1 Reagents and solutions

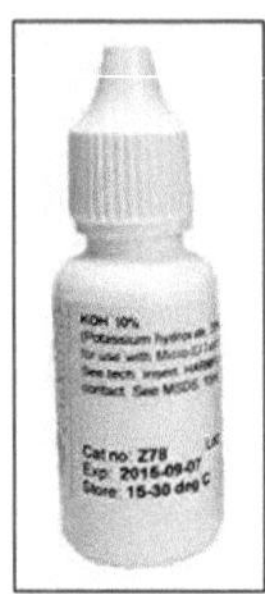

Figure 18: Potassium hydroxide KOH

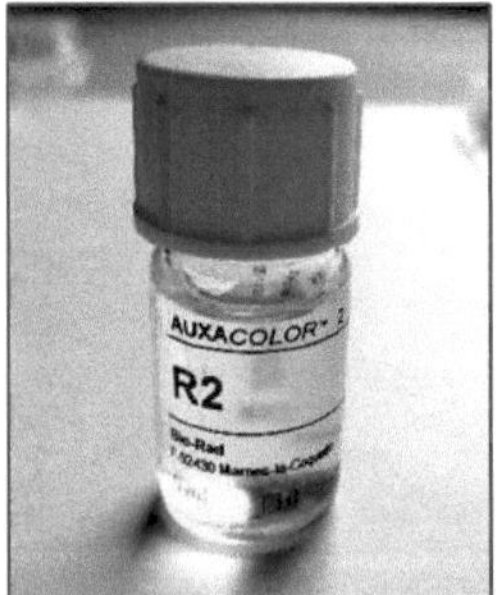

Figure 19: Auxacolor suspension media

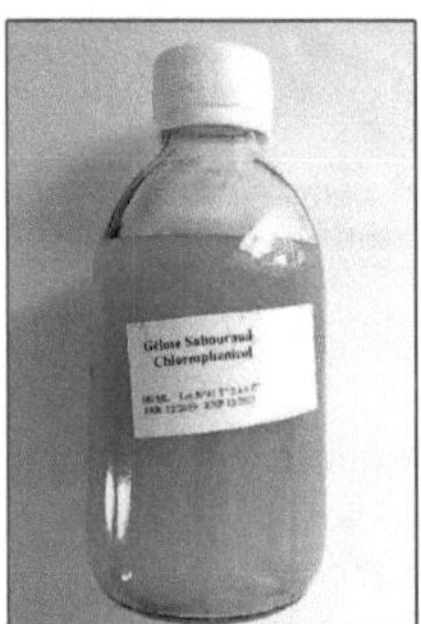

Figure 20: Sabouraud-Chloramphenicol agar bottle

1.6.2 Equipment for sampling

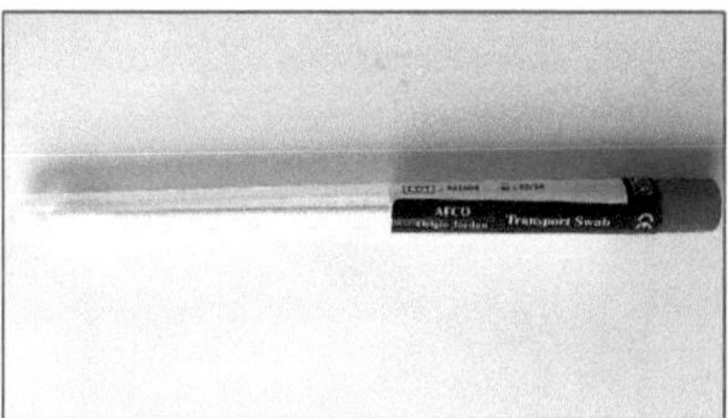

Figure 21: Sterile cotton swab

1.6.3 culture media

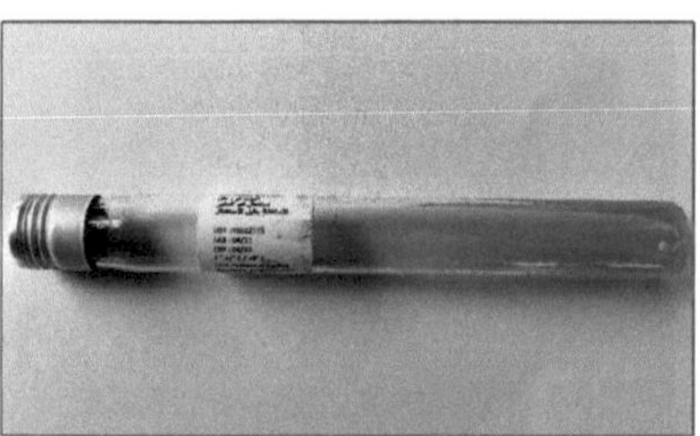

Figure 22: Sabouraud-chloramphenicol culture medium in tube

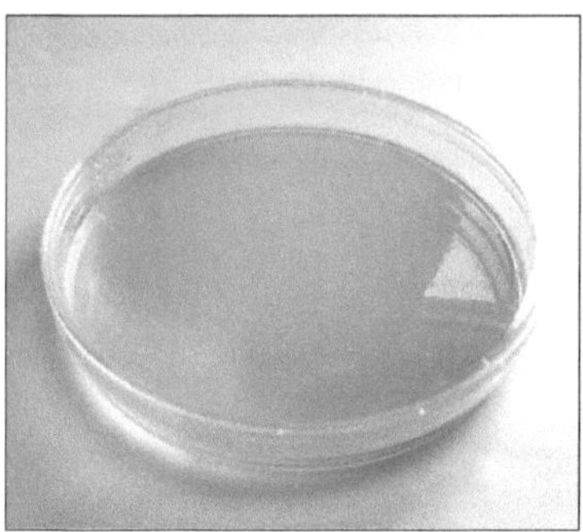

Figure 23: Sabouraud-chloramphenicol culture medium in petri dish

1.6.4 Equipment

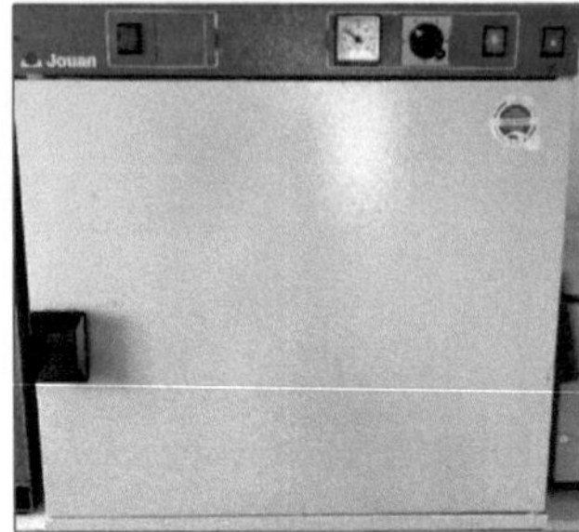

Figure 24: Oven at 37°C

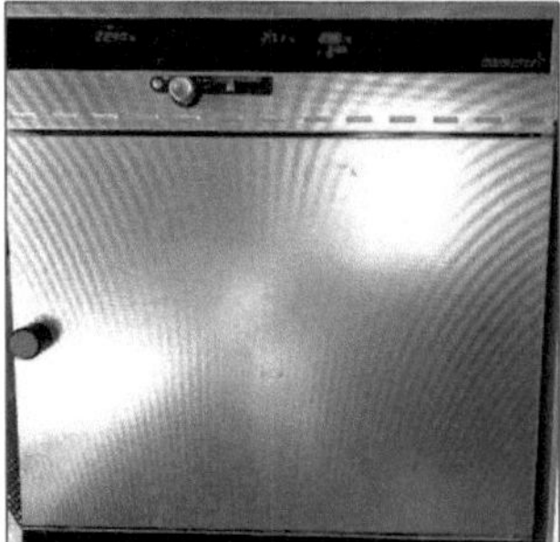

Figure 25: Oven at 27 °C

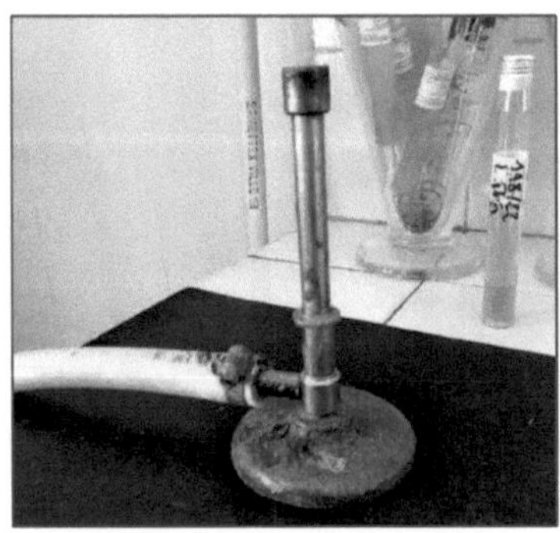

Figure 26.Bunsen burner

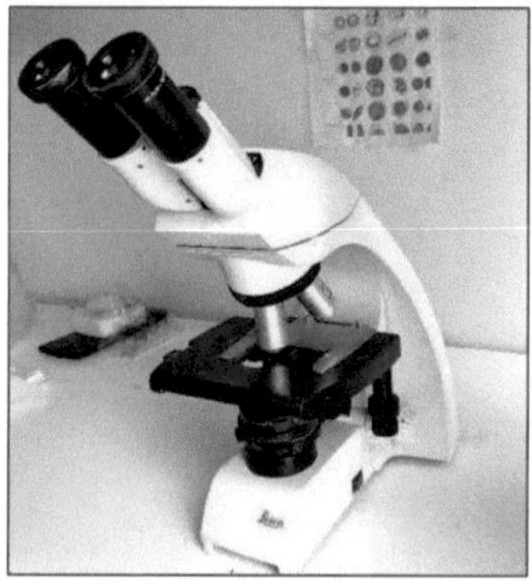

Figure 27: Optical microscope

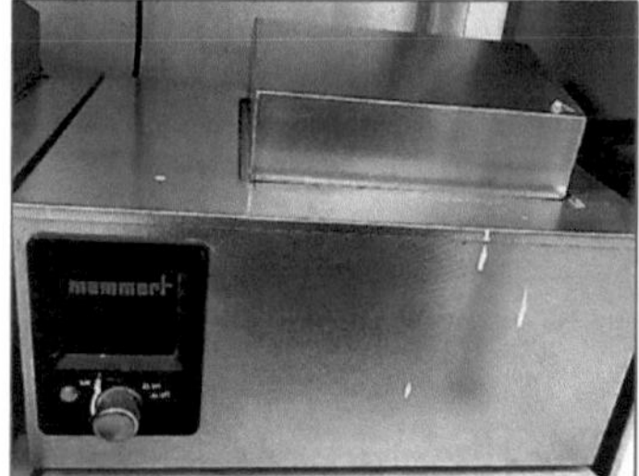

Figure 28: Water bath

1.6.5 Identification material

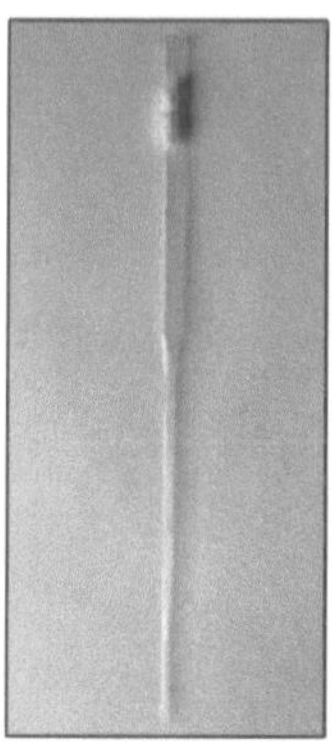

Figure 29: Glass pasteur pipette

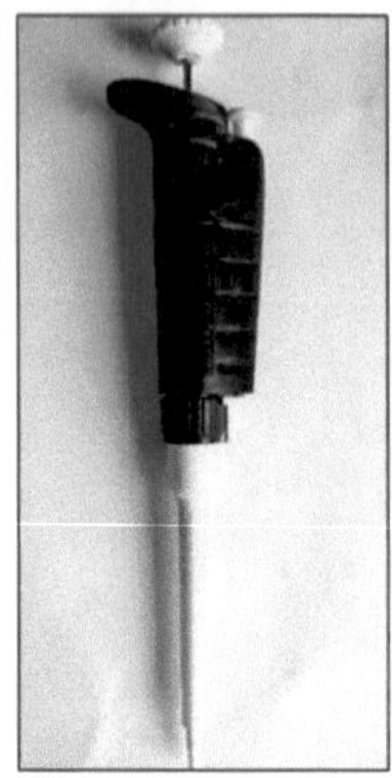

Figure 30: Piston pipette

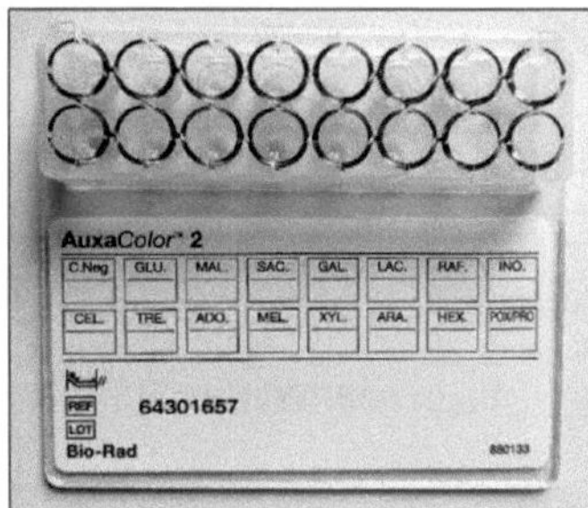

Figure 31: Auxacolor microplate

1.6.6 Other equipment consumables

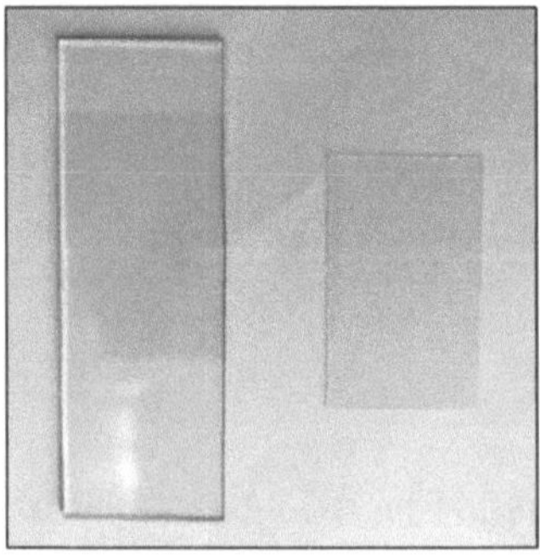

Figure 32: Blade and slat

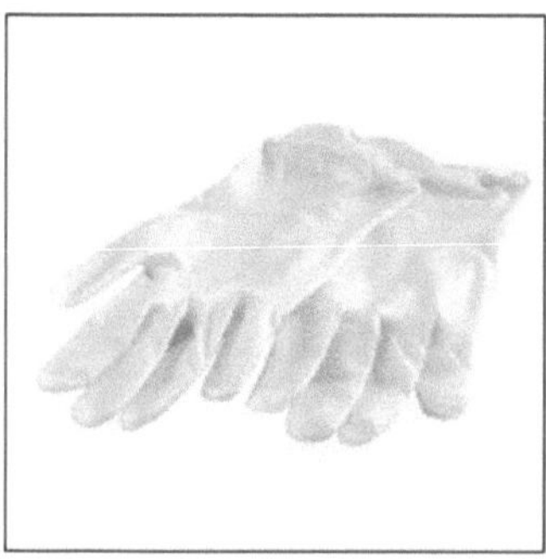

Figure 33: Gloves

2. Methodology

2.1 Sampling and examination

The clinical examination consists of looking for any changes in the oral mucosa, tongue, soft and hard palate, cheeks, periodontium and oropharynx, and any abnormal appearance of the mouth (whitish patches or coatings, redness, oral aphthosis, fissure of the tongue, dryness, inflammation, erythema of the tissues covered by the prosthesis, fissure and crusting of the labial commissures, etc.).After a thorough oral examination of the entire oral cavity, sterile swabs were taken from the tongue, the inside of the cheeks, the soft palate or an identified lesion.Samples were taken preferably on an empty stomach, in a sterile environment, and then analysed.forwarded as soon as possible to the parasitology and medical mycology department. A total of 78 samples were taken during our study.

2.2 Preparation of culture media

Under sterile conditions, petri dishes were poured with a sufficient quantity Sabouraud chloramphenicol agar, which had previously been melted in a water bath.After the agar has solidified, a number of petri dishes are subjected to a test ofsterility in the 37° oven to control the quality of the media. The culture media are then stored in the refrigerator.

2.3 Mycological culture

Before inoculating the samples, all sterile conditions were maintained and the culture tubes were numbered. Near the Bunsen burner, the samples were cultured in Sabouraud medium with added chloramphenicol, and then incubated in an oven at 37°C for 24 to 48 hours.

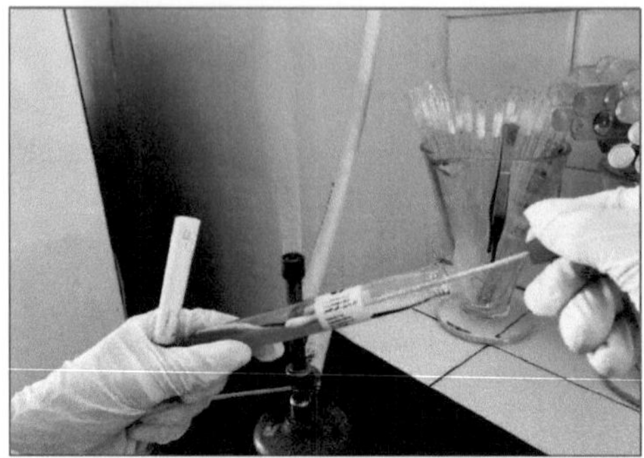

Figure 34: Inoculation of buccal swabs into culture media.

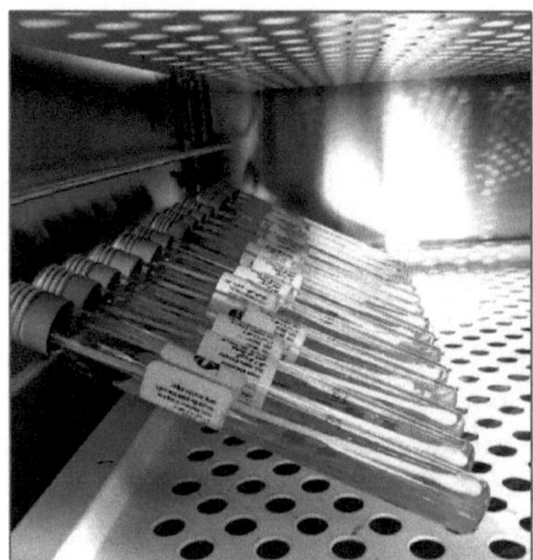

Figure 35: Incubation culture media in the oven at 37°C for 48 hours.

2.4 Macroscopic examination

Examination with the naked eye can differentiate the appearance of the colonies; a positive result is revealed by the presence of creamy-white colonies a few millimetres in diameter with smooth, shiny surfaces and sometimes dry, matt or wrinkled surfaces.

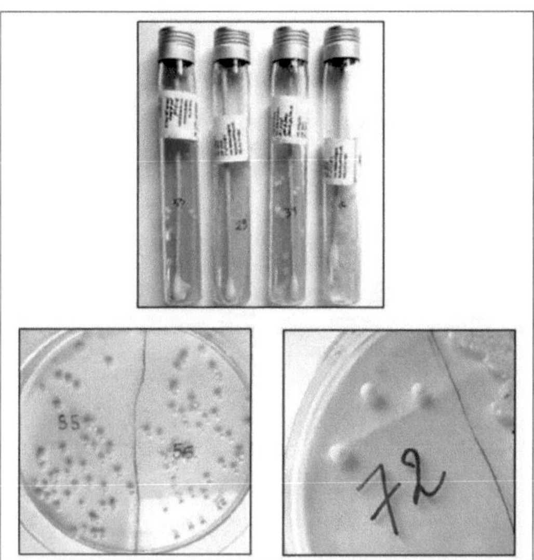

Figure 36: Macroscopic aspects of positive cultures on sabouraud media chlormaphenicol after 48 hours incubation at 37°C

2.5 Examination microscopic

The colonies resulting from the culture can be examined between slide and coverslip and with the addition of drops of KOH, spherical or ovoid yeasts, budded or not, a few micrometres in diameter, can be seen under the light microscope.

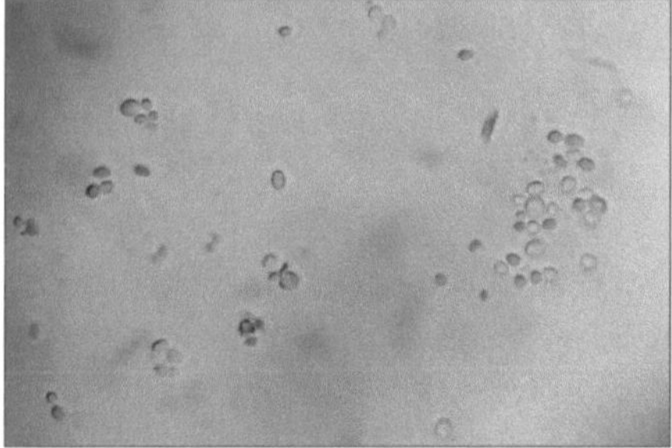

Figure 37: Direct examination of colonies after culture under a light microscope

2.6 Identifying the Auxacolor species

After 48 h incubation at 27°C of 100 µl of a suspension containing colonies of pure strains in microplate wells, the change in colour of each well helps in interpretation of positive and negative reactions, then coding system is established. The final identification of the species is based on a combination of biochemical tests and additional characteristics (morphological and metabolic) determined under the usual conditions (see appendices 2 and 3).

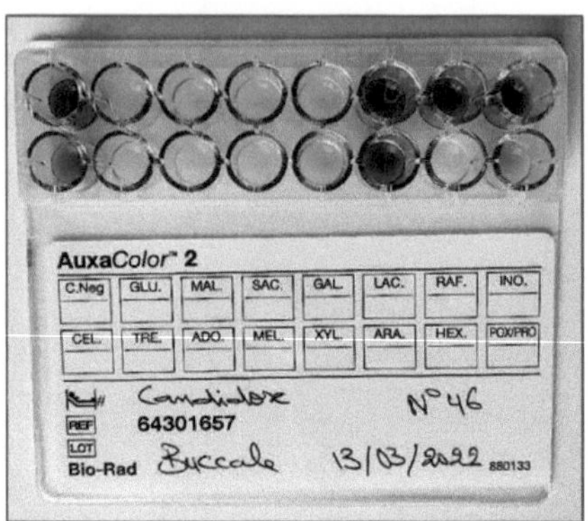

Figure 38.AUXACOLOR microplate after 48h incubation at 27°C

RESULTS

1.The prevalence of oral candidiasis in diabetic patients

- During the study period, 78 diabetic patients were included in our study, including 49 patients (63%) with proven oral candidiasis. (Figure 39)

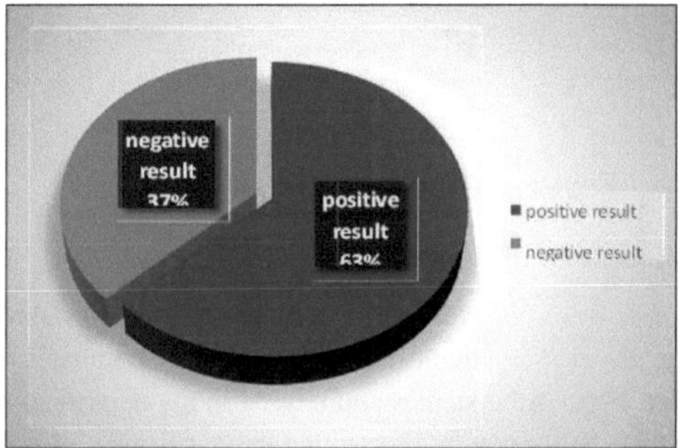

Figure 39: Prevalence of oral candidiasis in patients included in the study.the study

2. Breakdown of patients by age

- The 0-15 age group was the most representative, accounting for 40% of cases. (Figure 40).

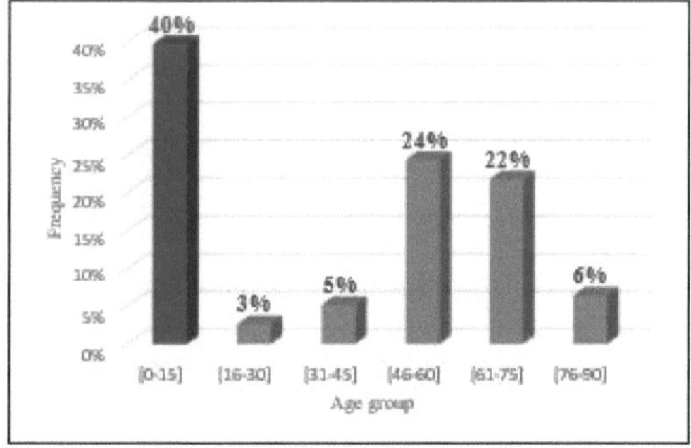

Figure 40.Breakdown of patients age

3. Breakdown of patients by sex

- We noted the predominance of males, 41 men (53%) compared with females, 37 women (47%). (Figure 41).

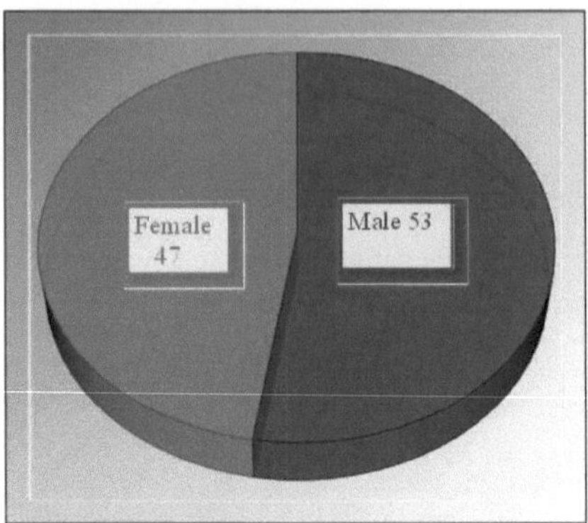

Figure 41: Breakdown of patients by sex

4. Breakdown of patients by hospital

▪ The majority of patients were hospitalised in the paediatrics department with a frequency of 40%, followed by the internal medicine department with frequency of 31%. The lowest frequency was recorded in the orthopaedics and traumatology department (9%).
▪ Our study revealed that the frequency of positive cases of oral candidiasis was higher than negative cases of oral candidiasis, regardless of the department. (Table 2)

Table 2.Breakdown all patients by hospital

Service	Result+		Result -		Total	
	Workforce	Percentage %	Workforce	Percentage %	Workforce	Percentage %
Paediatrics	19	61%	12	39%	31	40%
Medicine internal	16	67%	8	33%	24	31%
Orthopaedics and Traumatology	4	57%	3	43%	7	9%
Cardiology	10	63%	6	38%	16	21%
Total	49	63%	29	37%	78	100%

5. Breakdown of positive cases by tooth brushing habits

▪ Among patients with proven oral candidiasis, 61% are in the habit of to brush their teeth. (Figure 42)

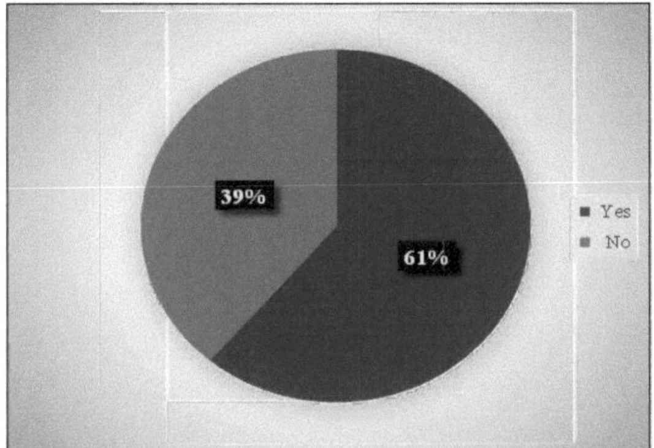

Figure 42: Breakdown of positive cases by tooth brushing habits

6. Breakdown of positive cases according to visits to the dentist

- Of the 49 patients with oral candidiasis, 73% did not have consulted a dentist for a long . (Figure 43)

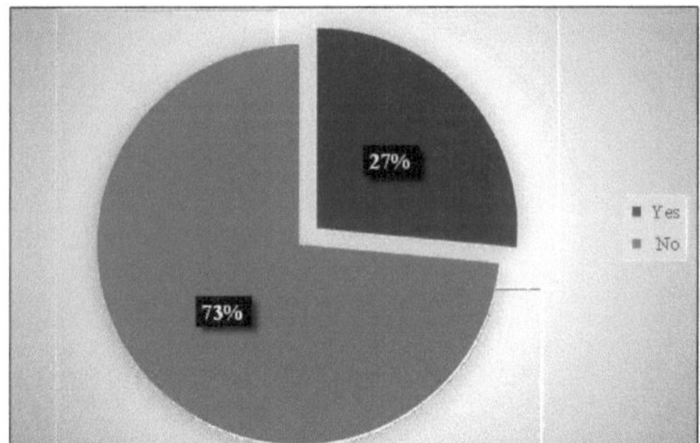

Figure 43: Breakdown of positive cases according to consultation with a dentist

7. Breakdown of positive cases by type of diabetes

- We noted that 59% of cases of oral candidiasis were linked to type II diabetes (Figure 44).

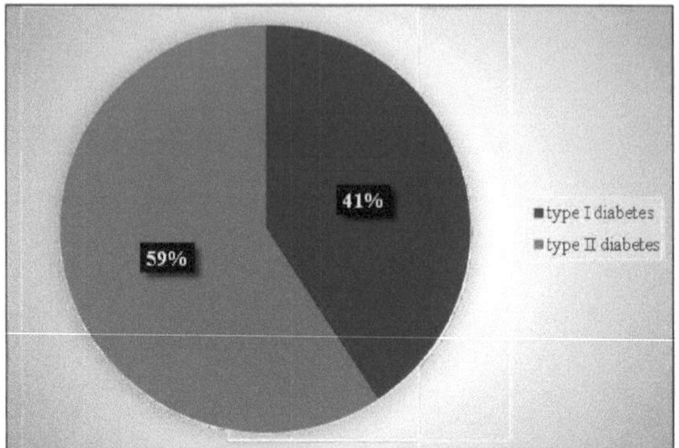

Figure 44: Breakdown positive cases by type of diabetes

8. Breakdown of positive cases according to whether or not diabetes is controlled

- Of all the patients with proven oral candidiasis, 90% had unbalanced diabetes with disturbed blood glucose levels above 1.26 g/l. (Figure 45)

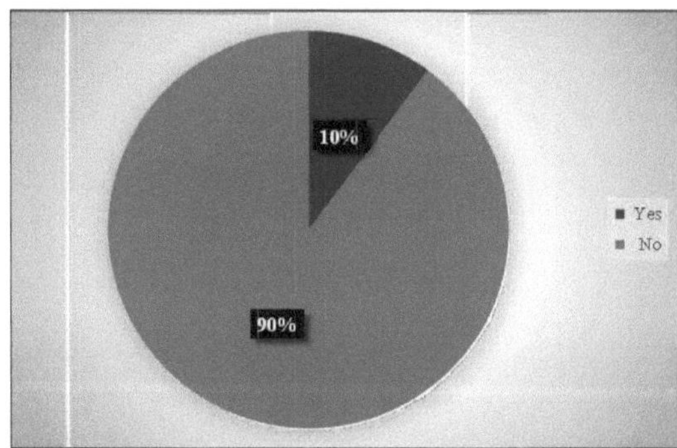

Figure 45: Distribution of positive cases according diabetes control

9. Breakdown of positive cases by reason for hospitalisation

- Diabetic ketoacidosis and acute coronary syndrome were the most common reasons for hospitalisation in our patients, with frequencies of 39% and 20% respectively.
- The other reasons for hospitalisation (diabetic foot, digestive haemorrhage, fracture and trauma, liver disease and thrombosis) were almost equally frequent.
- Renal disease was the least reason hospitalisation. (Figure 46)

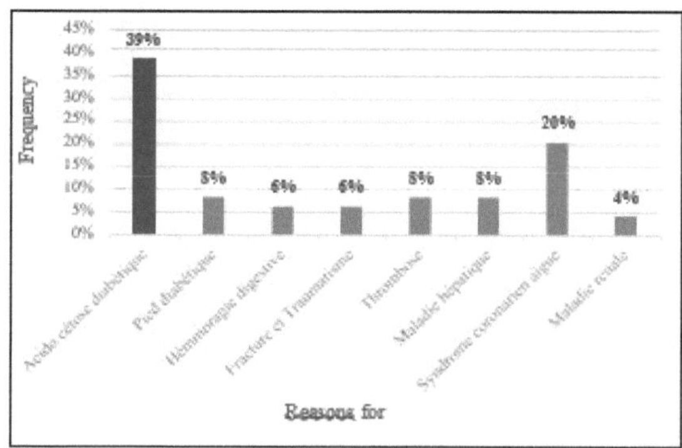

Figure 46: Breakdown of positive cases by reason for hospitalisation

10. Distribution of positive cases according to clinical form

▪ Our study revealed that among patients with oral candidiasis, 23 had a normal appearance of the mouth.
▪ In the rest of our patients, thrush and mouth ulcers were the most common clinical forms.
▪ Sometimes several aspects are identified in the same patient. (Figure 47)

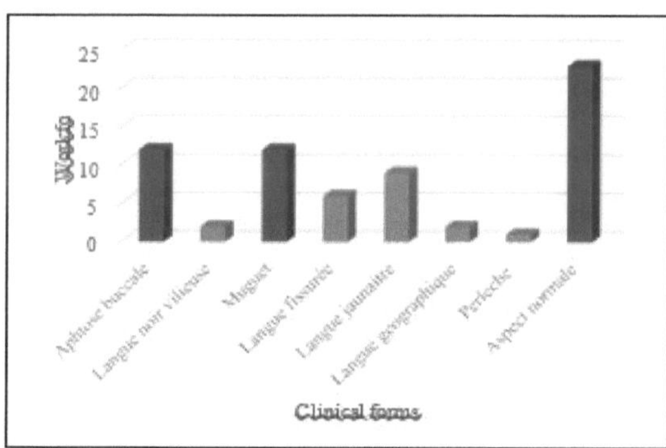

Figure 47: Distribution of positive cases according to clinical form

11. Distribution of positive cases according to medical and surgical history

▪ Hypertension the most common medical history (18 cases), followed by liver disease (8 cases).
▪ The rest of the antecedents are detailed in (Figure 48).

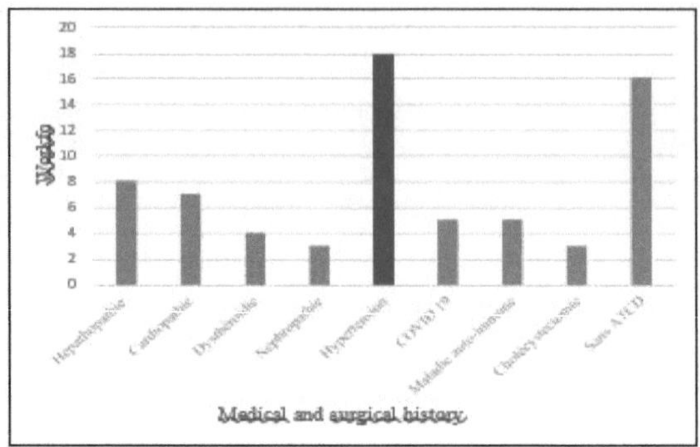

Figure 48: Distribution of positive cases according to medical and surgical history

12. Breakdown of positive cases according to treatment received

- Of the diabetic patients with oral candidiasis, 42 were using insulin therapy.
- Other patients take oral antidiabetic drugs either alone or in combination. in association with insulin therapy.
- Cardiology drugs, anticoagulants and antibiotics are among the classes of drugs most used by our patients. (Figure 49).

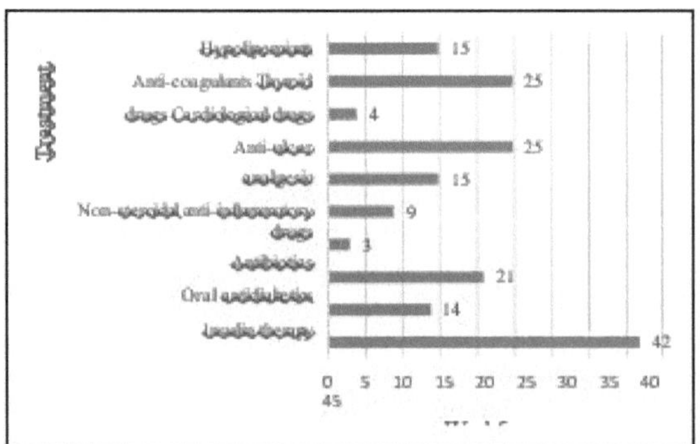

Figure 49: Distribution of positive cases according to treatment received

- 21 patients were treated with antibiotics. Betalactam antibiotics were the most commonly used class ATBs (67%). (Figure 50)

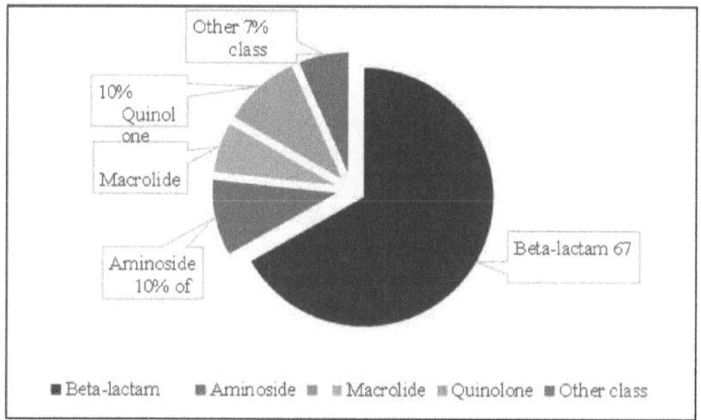

Figure 50.Breakdown of patients by class of antibiotics used

13. Breakdown of positive cases according to risk factors

- The most common risk factor for oral candidiasis was antibiotic therapy (26%), followed by diabetic ketoacidosis (24%) and dentures (15%).
- The other factors are detailed in (Figure 51).

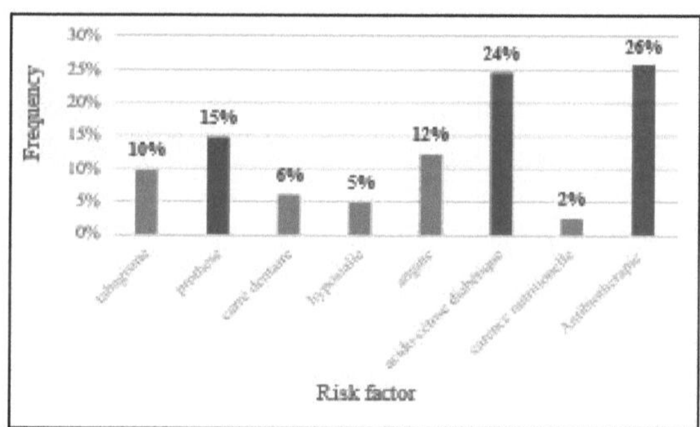

Figure 51: Distribution of positive cases according to risk factors

14. Breakdown of positive cases by Candida species

- We obtained 49 positive cultures.

- Candida albicans was the most frequently isolated species with a frequency 37%, followed by Candida dubliniensis with a frequency of 27%, and Candida tropicalis with a frequency of 18%. (Figure 52)

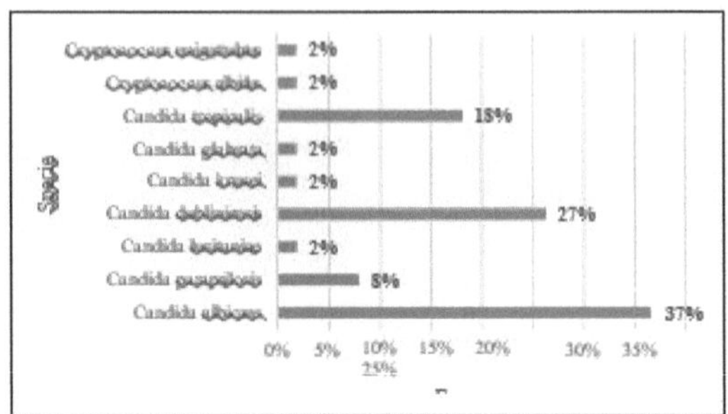

Figure 52: Breakdown of positive cases by species

15. Results of mycological culture and identification of each species

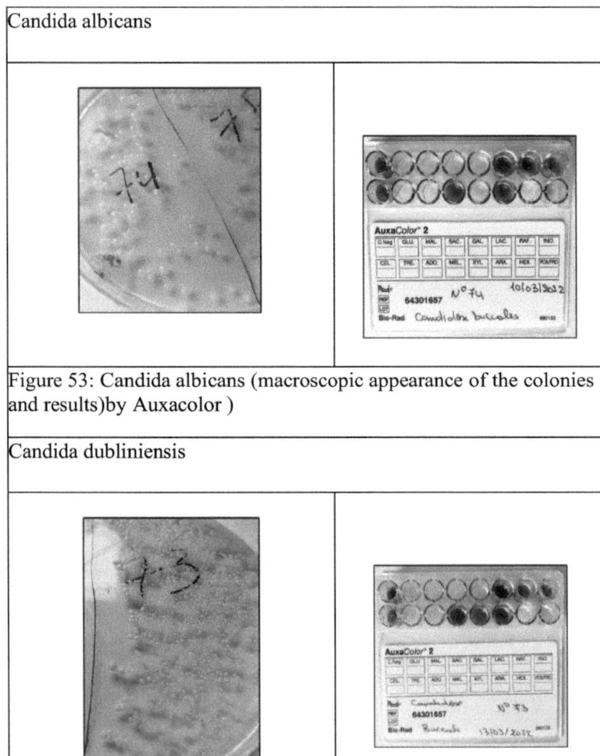

Candida albicans

Figure 53: Candida albicans (macroscopic appearance of the colonies and results)by Auxacolor)

Candida dubliniensis

Figure 54.Candida dubliniensis (macroscopic appearance of colonies and resultsby Auxacolor)

Candida tropicalis	
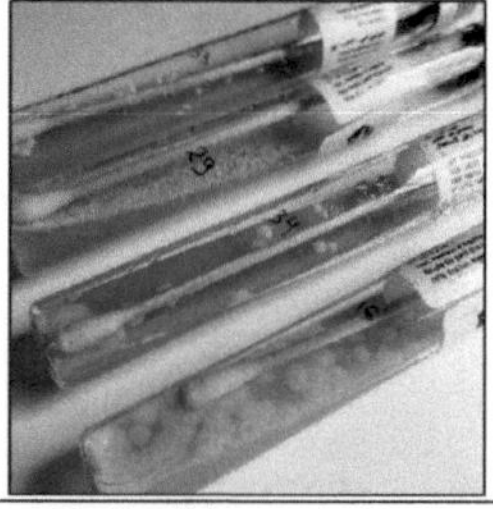	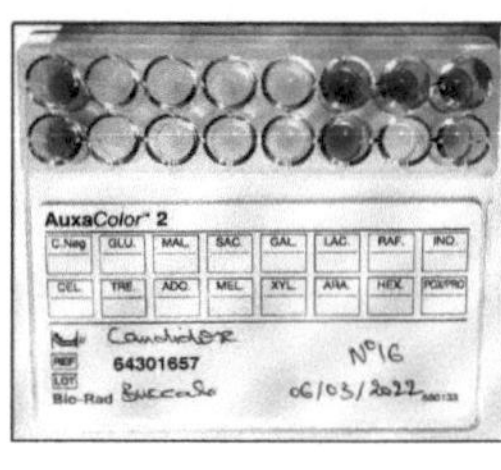
Figure 55.Candida tropicalis (macroscopic appearance of colonies and results by Auxacolor)	
Candida parapsilosis	
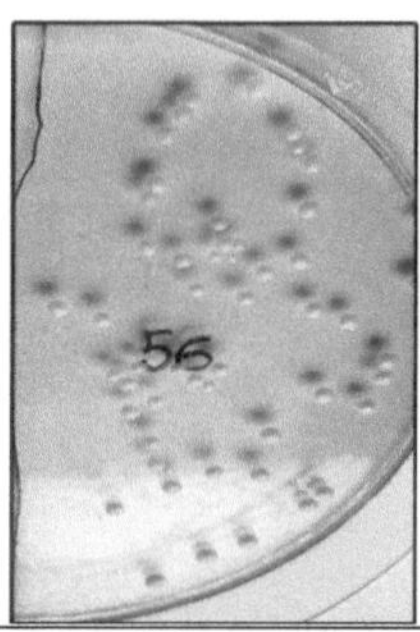	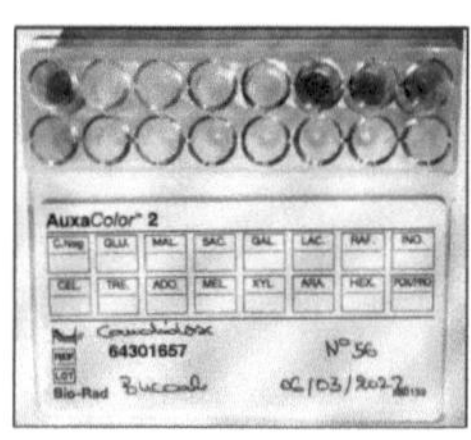
Figure 56.Candida parapsilosis (macroscopic appearance of colonies and results by Auxacolor)	

Candida lusitaniae

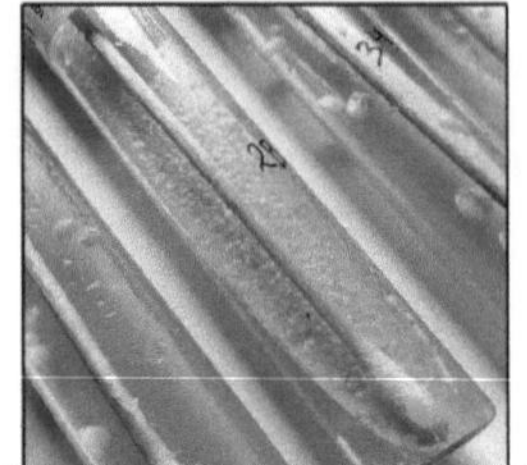

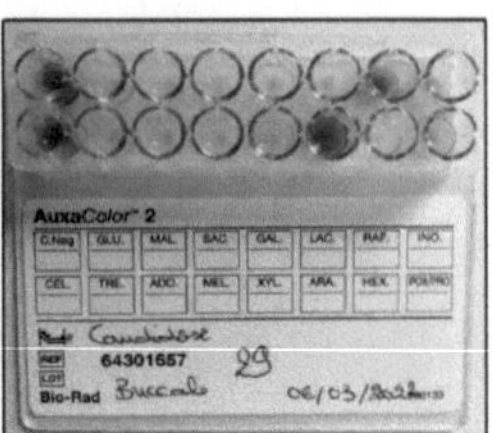

Figure 57.Candida luisitaniae (macroscopic appearance of colonies and results by Auxacolor)

Candida krusei

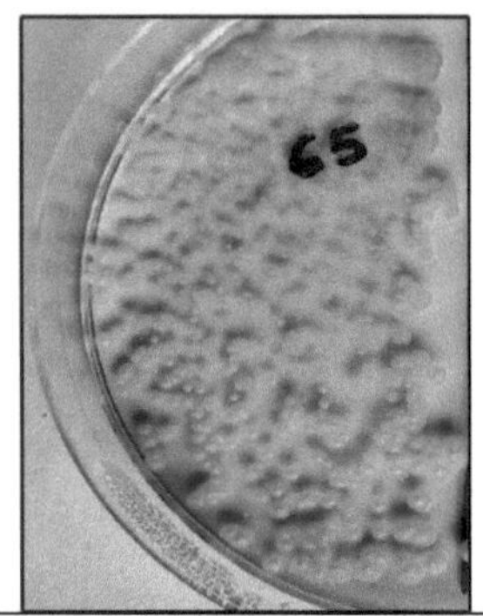

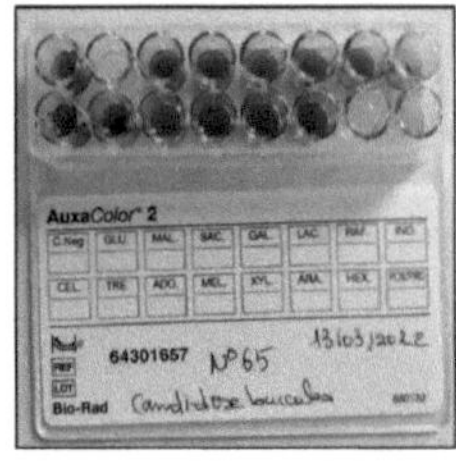

Figure 58: Candida krusei (macroscopic appearance of the colonies and results) by Auxacolor)

Candida glabrata	
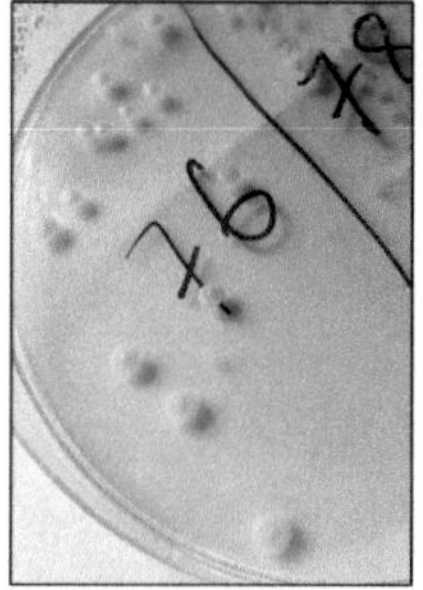	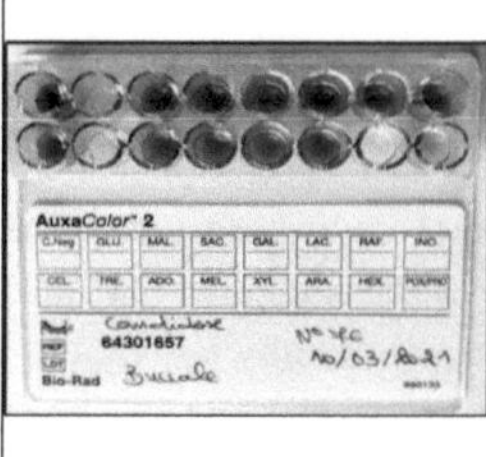
Figure 59: Candida glabrata (macroscopic appearance of the colonies and results)by Auxacolor)	
Cryptococcus albidus	
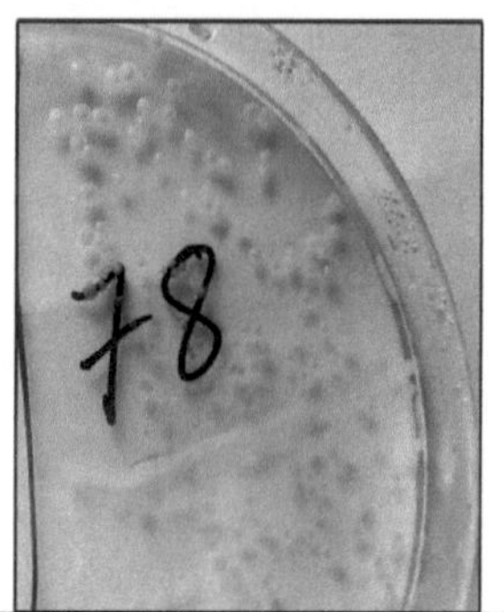	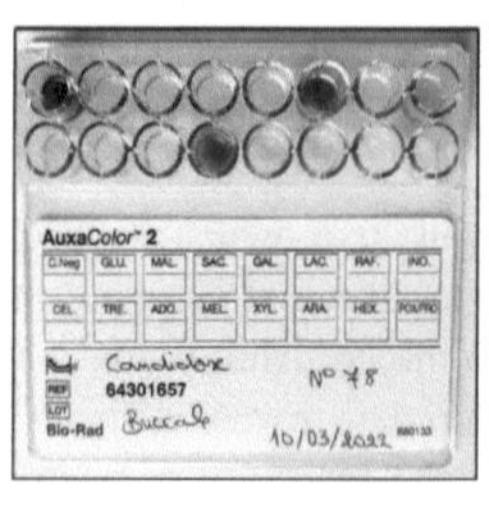
Figure 60.Cryptococcus albidus (macroscopic appearance of colonies and results by Auxacolor)	
Cryptococcus uniguttulatus	
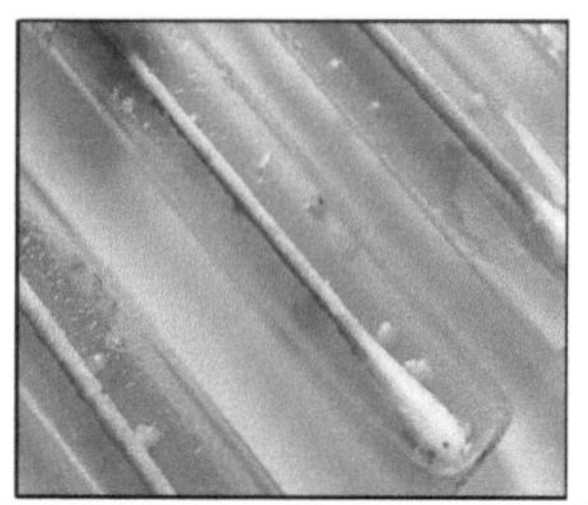	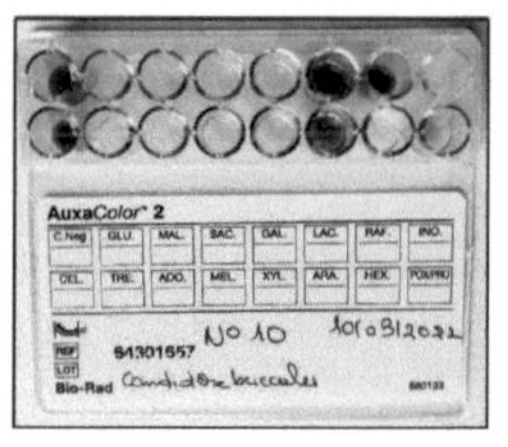
Figure 61.Cryptococcus uniguttulatus (macroscopic appearance of the colonies and result Auxacolor)	

DISCUSSION

Diabetes is a chronic disease that is widespread the world and has an impact on the daily lives of millions of people. The general weakness of the immune system and poor glycaemic control make DM patients more vulnerable to the development secondary infections. Infections of the oral cavity are very common in DM patients, oral candidiasis being one them. Previous research suggests that the risk of developing oral candidiasis is higher in people with DM than in healthy individuals due to a variety of contributing factors [2].

The aim of our study was to determine the prevalence of BC in diabetic patients and the species involved. We also aimed to describe the risk factors for the occurrence of BC. The prevalence of oral candidiasis in our patients was 63%, a result very similar to that found in the study by Belazi et al, in 2005, who found a frequency of 64% of oral candidiasis in diabetic subjects, and 40% in healthy subjects [50]. Another result is that Mohammadi et al, in 2016, who found a 55% frequency of oral candidiasis in diabetic patients [28]. The age range [0-15 years] was the most represented with 40% of cases, our result is far from that found by Adiaratou walet hamed saleh, during a study on the epidemio-clinical aspects of lesions of the oral mucosa in 266 diabetic patients at the Mali hospital in 2019, where the age range between [10-25 years] was the most representative with frequency of 42.90% of cases [51].

In our study, the majority of patients were male (53%), a result close to that of the study by Mohammadi et al in 2016, which showed that 65.5% of patients were male [28]. This can be explained by a lack hygiene (brushing the teeth), the consumption of alcohol or drugs, or a lack of hygiene. tobacco. And during our study period we found more men in hospital than women.women.Our data revealed that Candida albicans species was the most frequently isolated from the oral cavity (37%), which is in line with the results found in the study by Mohammadi et al in Iran in 2016 who found a similar result 36.2% [28]. Candida albicans has the ability to adhere to mucosal and denture surfaces, which is considered the first step in pathogenesis, The ability of Candida albicans to respond to changes in the host environment can respond to the increase in the number of colony forming units, and invade tissues and cause infections that require the spread of intimacy of care due cooperation with the denture [52]. Candida dubliniensis was the non-albicans species most frequently found (27%). Our result is consistent with that found by Mamari et al in Yemen in 2017 with a frequency of (17%) for the same species [52]. We also noted the emergence of new species such as: (Candida parapsilosis, Candida lusitaniae, Candida krusei, Candida glabrata,); as well as Cryptococcus albidus and Cryptococcus uniguttulatus). Recently, the infectious potential of non-albicans Candida species in the oral cavity has received increased attention. This has also been exacerbated by the COVID-19 pandemic, as an increase in oral candidiasis has been observed [53].

The identification of these species has become important because they differ both in their potential to cause disease and in their response to antifungal agents [54]. Many pathogenicity factors in Candida spp have been attributed to the increased incidence of candidiasis in diabetic patients, such as enzymatic activity, biofilm formation, hydrophobicity, phenotype change and yeast-hyphal transition. The production of extracellular enzymes by Candida spp may play an important role in its pathogenicity, invasion, destruction of host tissues and onset of clinical signs. Candida spp also use their enzymes phospholipase and esterase to invade host tissues and haemolysin to lyse blood cells. Although Candida has the ability to produce these enzymes, the quantity and strength of these enzymes vary from species to species, and because of the different sources of their isolation, they have different modes of secretion. Phospholipase secretions also help the organism to penetrate host tissues more effectively [1].

The pathogenic capacity of Candida species and their colonisation factors depend on host-related immune factors due to a complex homeostatic relationship between the fungi and the host's current immune status. Predisposition to the creation an environment conducive to Candida multiplication include various factors such as reduced intestinal secretions, dietary causes, altered gastrointestinal microflora, immunosuppression and concomitant diseases, continuous use of ATBs or other drugs, altered liver function and a lack of necessary nutrients [2].

Our study found that several factors favour the onset of the disease in this category, including diabetic imbalance, which is one of the major factors involved in the disease, and we found that 90% of cases of BC involve patients with disturbed blood sugar levels, as well as diabetic ketoacidosis, which is the most frequent reason for hospitalisation (39%).

This was in agreement with studies by Khosravi et al in 2008 and Al Moubarak et al in 2013 who stated that the degree of Candida prevalence in the oral cavity can be modified by blood glucose levels. This finding may explain that a high carbohydrate diet or poor glycaemic control in diabetic patients can promote Candida overgrowth and increase the production of hydrolytic enzymes, such as secreted aspartyl proteases (SAPs) and phospholipases (LPs), These enzymes not only promote yeast invasion of the altered oral epithelium, but also offer direct cytotoxicity and induce the inflammation of the mucosa observed in atrophic or erythematous candidiasis [49,55,56] .

The use of high doses and long duration of antibiotic therapy was the most common risk factor, particularly during the COVID-19 pandemic, implicated in the development of oral candidiasis. In our study, a large number of patients consumed antibiotics, mainly beta-lactam antibiotics (67%), a result similar to ours was found by Vijay et al. in 2021 in INDIA, during a study of secondary infections in hospitalised patients with COVID-19 [57], 16% of our patients presented with angina, making it necessary to prescribe TBAs. Another study by Salehi et al in 2020 in Iran found that out of 53 cases of COVID-19 hospitalized with oropharyngeal candidiasis where cardiovascular disease and diabetes were the most common underlying conditions in addition to other risk factors such as old age, admission to intensive care, lymphocytopenia Broad-spectrum antibiotics and corticosteroids are used to treat hypertension. observed in our patients of 26%, followed by acute coronary syndrome [58].
The microenvironment of the denture-bearing palatal mucosa is poorly oxygenated, largely devoid of saliva and has a low acid pH, which may favour the hydrolytic enzymatic activity of Candida virulence, Thus, the risk of contracting oral candidiasis was significantly higher in diabetics wearing dentures than in those who did not. In our study of 15 diabetic patients wearing dentures, 12 (80%) had BC [49]. In terms of oral hygiene, most of our patients brushed their teeth, although there was a significant prevalence of BC, which can be

explained by differences in the frequency, timing and technique of brushing.It has also been noted that diabetics are more prone to the accumulation of debris and calculus, despite having similar oral hygiene habits to non-diabetics. This may be due to the fact that excess glucose reaches the oral cavity via saliva and gingival crevicular fluid in patients with poor metabolic control, and contributes to a sugar-rich biofilm, which enhances plaque and tartar growth, in our study a percentage 6% presenting with dental squares having a BC [59]. In addition, tobacco smoking is considered to be the most important risk factor in the development of multiple pathological conditions of the oral mucosa, in particular oral candidiasis, with a significant percentage of 10% of our population having BC.Most of our patients had asymptomatic oral candidiasis revealed by a positive culture (34%). The clinical forms most frequently observed are: acute pseudomembranous disease (thrush) 18%, oral aphthosis 18%, yellowish tongue 13% and cracked tongue 9%. Geographic tongue, black tongue and perlèche are rare in our population.

CONCLUSION AND OUTLOOK

Diabetes is a chronic disease considered to be one of the main causes of illness and premature death in most countries. It is a major problem worldwide, with multiple co-morbidities and huge economic losses for patients, their families and healthcare systems, including lost productivity and pressure on national economies. It also increases the risk of systemic and oral complications, particularly oral candidiasis.Oral candidiasis is the fungal infection most frequently encountered in diabetic patients, caused mainly by a yeast of the genus Candida. Although Candida is a normal commensal of the oral cavity, a number of factors can predispose to the occurrence of BC, including extreme age, hyperglycaemia, immune dysfunction, underlying diseases such as heart disease, hypertension, liver disease, dysthyroidism, infectious diseases linked to the increased use of long-term antibiotic therapy, particularly for angina and covid 19. Inadequate oral hygiene, smoking, the use of dental prostheses a The presence of dental caries over a long period of time is also a contributing factor.The aim of our work was establish the specific prevalence of oral candidiasis in diabetics, identify the species involved and to determine the favourable risk factors based on focused questioning and mycological diagnosis. Mycological diagnosis is based on the culture of samples in specific media, direct examination of colonies and, finally, identification of the species important for the correct choice of treatment. Systemic health is linked to oral health, particularly in people with diabetes, which increases the need for dental and medical management of the patient. To improve the general and oral health of diabetic patients, a collaborative relationship between patients, pharmacists, doctors and dentists needs to be developed. Many patients with diabetes are unaware of the relationship between their disease and oral health. So the involvement of healthcare professionals in strategies for recognising, preventing and screening for the disease have become essential. The following preventive measures and recommendations are therefore proposed:

Diabetic patients

- Encourage diabetic patients to see their dentist at least twice a year for a routine check-up, and thus to obtain more information on oral health.
- Make patients aware that oral pathologies can be a cause of diabetes complications.
- Educating parents about the oral health of their diabetic children.
- The internet can be used to educate DM patients because of its increasing use.
- Motivating patients to eat healthy foods, reduce body weight and manage blood pressure, cholesterol levels, emotional problems and physical activity.

Dentists

- Better treatment results can be achieved if dental practitioners are aware of the dental complications and risk factors of DM.
- Providing advice to diabetic patients on the use of fluoride mouthwash, brushing teeth with fluoride toothpaste twice a day and flossing once a day should be encouraged to ensure plaque

control.

o Advise patients with dentures to remove them at night and adjust the denture incorrectly with regular use of antimicrobial cleansers.

Doctors

o Updating information and educational material on oral health.

o Organise campaigns and educational activities to raise awareness among people with diabetes about oral health and oral complications, particularly candidiasis.

o Early identification, assessment and management of diabetic patients.

o Include an oral and dental check-up as part of diabetes management assessments.

o Mycological examination is often ignored in the care of diabetic patientswhich is why needs to be introduced for better management.

Pharmacists

o Promote and support research that will lead to evidence-based treatment strategies to improve the health of diabetic patients

o Advising patients on the correct use of medication and glycaemic control in order to reduce the complications associated with imbalance

o Assess the severity of the infection before recommending drugs for sale free.

ETHICS AND LIMITATIONS

Ethics

Free and informed consent was obtained from each patient before the examination by means of a detailed explanation of our study, professional secrecy was safeguarded, and confidentiality and anonymity were de rigueur. Ethical principles (respect for patients, beneficence, etc.) were respected. The study took account of good medical practice.

Limitation

The number of patients with clinical signs and symptoms of oral candidiasis was very low compared to previous studies.

BIBLIOGRAPHICAL REFERENCE

1. Nouraei H, Jahromi MG, Jahromi LR, Zomorodian K, Pakshir K. Potential Pathogenicity of Candida Species Isolated from Oral Cavity of Patients with Diabetes Mellitus. Garg H, editor. BioMed Res Int. 2021;2021:1- 6.

2. Mohammed L, Jha G, Malasevskaia I, Goud HK, Hassan A. The Interplay Between Sugar and Yeast Infections: Do Diabetics Have a Greater Predisposition to Develop Oral and Vulvovaginal Candidiasis? Cureus. 13(2):e13407.

3. Rodrigues CF, Rodrigues ME, Henriques M. Candida sp. Infections in Patients with Diabetes Mellitus. J Clin Med. 2019;8(1):76.

4. R AN, Rafiq NB. Candidiasis. In: StatPearls [Internet]. Treasure Island (FL): StatPearls Publishing; 2022 [cited 2022 Mar 11]. Available from: http://www.ncbi.nlm.nih.gov/books/NBK560624/

5. Szabo EK, MacCallum DM. The contribution of mouse models to our understanding of systemic candidiasis. FEMS Microbiol Lett. Jul 2011;320(1):1- 8.

6. Marieb EN, Hoehn K, Moussakova L, Lachaine R. Human anatomy and physiology. 9 th edition. Montreuil: Pearson; 2015.

7. Drake RL, Vogl W, Mitchell AWM, Duparc F, Duparc J. Gray's anatomy for students. 2nd edition. Issy-les-Moulineaux: Elsevier Masson; 2010.

8. Larousse É. oral mucosa - LAROUSSE [Internet]. [cited 24 Feb 2022]. Available from: https://www.larousse.fr/encyclopedie/medical/muqueuse_buccale/14654

9. Auriol M, charpentier M. Histology of the buccal mucosa and maxillae. Encycl Méd Chir (Elsevier, Paris), Stomatology;22-007-M-10,1998,9p.

10. Grandgirard F. Consequences of hormonal pathologies on the oral mucosa [Thesis]. NANCY Univ HENRI POINCARE. 2002;

11. Moris DV, Melhem MSC, Martins MA, Mendes RP. Oral Candida spp. colonization in human immunodeficiency virus-infected individuals. J Venom Anim Toxins Trop Dis. 2008;14(2):224- 57.

12. Singh A, Verma R, Murari A, Agrawal A. Oral candidiasis: An overview. J Oral Maxillofac Pathol JOMFP. Sep 2014;18(Suppl 1):S81- 5.

13. Ciurea CN, Kosovski IB, Mare AD, Toma F, Pintea-Simon IA, Man A. Candida and Candidiasis-Opportunism Versus Pathogenicity: A Review of the Virulence Traits. Microorganisms. 2020;8(6):857.

14. Koenig H. Guide de mycologie médicale. Paris: Ellipses; 1995.

15. Ripert C. Mycologie médicale. 2013e ed. Paris: Lavoisier; 218- 219 p.

16. Talapko J, Juzbašić M, Matijević T, Pustijanac E, Bekić S, Kotris I, et al. Candida albicans-The Virulence Factors and Clinical Manifestations of Infection. J Fungi. 2021;7(2):79 p.

17. Dufresne P. Identification des champignons d'importance médicale. 2021;1-64 p.

18. Dominique Chabasse, Raymond Robert, Agnès Marot, Marc Pihet. Candida pathogènes. Paris: Éd. Tec & doc; 2006. (Microbiology monographs).

19. Williams DW, Kuriyama T, Silva S, Malic S, Lewis MAO. Candida biofilms and oral candidosis: treatment and prevention: Candida biofilms and oral candidosis. Periodontol 2000. Feb 2011;55(1):250- 65.

20. Williams D, Lewis M. Pathogenesis and treatment of oral candidosis. J Oral Microbiol. 1 Jan 2011;3(1):5771.

21. Silva S, Negri M, Henriques M, Oliveira R, Williams DW, Azeredo J. Candida glabrata, Candida parapsilosis and Candida tropicalis: biology, epidemiology, pathogenicity and antifungal resistance. FEMS Microbiol Rev. 2012;36(2):288- 305.

22. SANOGO OM. Candidoses digestives chez les PVVIH au SMIT du CHU Point G: Aspects épidémiologique, clinique, étiologique et thérapeutique. PhD thesis. USTTB; 2021.

23. Hoppe JE. Treatment of oropharyngeal candidiasis and candidal diaper dermatitis in neonates and infants: review and reappraisal. Pediatr Infect Dis J. 1997;16(9):885- 94.

24. DE REPENTIGNY L, LEWANDOWSKI D, JOLICOEUR P. Immunopathogenesis of Oropharyngeal Candidiasis in Human Immunodeficiency Virus Infection. Clinical microbiology reviews. 2004;729- 59.

25. CDC. 1993 Revised Classification System for HIV Infection and Expanded Surveillance Case Definition for AIDS Among Adolescents and Adults [Internet]. [cited 28 March 2022]. Available at: https://www.cdc.gov/mmwr/preview/mmwrhtml/00018871.htm

26. Darwazeh AMG, Lamey PJ, Samaranayake LP, Macfarlane TW, Fisher BM, Macrury SM, et al. The relationship between colonisation, secretor status and in-vitro adhesion of Candida albicans to buccal epithelial cells from diabetics. J Med Microbiol. 1990;33(1):43- 9.

27. Tarçın BG. Oral Candidosis: Aetiology, Clinical Manifestations, Diagnosis and Management. Clin Exp Health Sci. 2011;1(2):140.

28. Mohammadi F, Javaheri M, Nekoeian S, Dehghan P. Identification of Candida species in the oral cavity of diabetic patients. Curr Med Mycol. June 2016;2(2):1- 7.

29. Born F. Oral candidiasis: a review of the literature. 2013 [cited 23 March 2022]; Available from: https://archive-ouverte.unige.ch/unige:27981

30. Laurent M, Gogly B, Tahmasebi F, Paillaud E. Oropharyngeal candidiasis in elderly patients. Gériatrie Psychol Neuropsychiatr Viellissement. 2011;9(1):21- 8.

31. Davies AN, Brailsford SR, Beighton D, Shorthose K, Stevens VC. Oral Candidosis in

Community-Based Patients with Advanced Cancer. J Pain Symptom Manage. 2008;35(5):508- 14.

32. Barbagallo AL. A STUDY OF SUBGINGIVAL MICROBIAL DIVERSITY IN DIABETIC PATIENTS. 2012;76.

33. Akpan A. Oral candidiasis. Postgrad Med J. 2002;78(922):455- 9.

34. Bornstein MM, Klingler K, Saxer UP, Walter C, Ramseier CA. Oral mucosal changes associated with smoking. 2006;116:1270- 4.

35. Sharma A. Oral candidiasis: An opportunistic infection: A review. Int J Appl Dent Sci. 2019;5(1):23- 7.

36. Hellstein JW, Marek CL. Candidiasis: Red and White Manifestations in the Oral Cavity. Head Neck Pathol. March 2019;13(1):25- 32.

37. Vila T, Sultan AS, Montelongo-Jauregui D, Jabra-Rizk MA. Oral Candidiasis: A Disease of Opportunity. J Fungi. 16 Jan 2020;6(1):15.

38. BELAHCEN EL OUALI R. ORAL CANDIDIASIS IN CHILDREN. [RABAT]: MOHAMMED V UNIVERSITY - FACULTY OF MEDICINE AND PHARMACY; 2016.

39. Guyon A, Gaultier F, Glass P. Median rhomboid glossitis: the essentials. Rev Odont Stomat. 2017;46:126- 33.

40. Title : THE SABURRAL LANGUAGE [Internet]. [cited 7 May 2022]. Available from: https://www.google.com/imgres

41. Eric Burge BMus, Siddharth Kogilwaimath MD. Tongue in cheek. CMAJ. 12 Jul 2021;193(27).

42. Coronado-Castellote L, Jimenez-Soriano Y. Clinical and microbiological diagnosis of oral candidiasis. J Clin Exp Dent. 2013;e279-86.

43. Garcia-Cuesta C, Sarrion-Perez Mg, Bagan Jv. Current treatment of oral candidiasis: A literature review. J Clin Exp Dent. 2014;6(5):e576- 82.

44. Ferreira E dos S, Rosalen PL, Benso B, de Cássia Orlandi Sardi J, Denny C, Alves de Sousa S, et al. The Use of Essential Oils and Their Isolated Compounds for the Treatment of Oral Candidiasis: A Literature Review. Khan M, editor. Evid Based Complement Alternat Med. 7 Jan 2021;1- 16.

45. Gheorghe DC, Niculescu AG, Bîrcă AC, Grumezescu AM. Biomaterials for the Prevention of Oral Candidiasis Development. Pharmaceutics. 27 May 2021;13(6):803.

46. National Association of Clinical Pharmacy Teachers, publisher. Clinical pharmacy and therapeutics. 4th ed. Issy-les-Moulineaux: Elsevier Masson; 2012.

47. Martins N, Ferreira ICFR, Barros L, Silva S, Henriques M. Candidiasis: Predisposing Factors, Prevention, Diagnosis and Alternative Treatment. Mycopathologia. June 2014;177(5-

6):223- 40.

48. Hatakka K, Ahola AJ, Yli-knuuttila H, Richardson M, Poussa T, Meurman JH, et al. a Randomized Controlled Trial- - in the ElderlyCandidaProbiotics Reduce the Prevalence of Oral Published by: 2007.

49. Lu SY. Oral Candidosis: Pathophysiology and Best Practice for Diagnosis, Classification, and Successful Management. J Fungi. 13 Jul 2021;7(7):555.

50. Belazi M, Velegraki A, Fleva A, Gidarakou I, Papanaum L, Baka D, et al. Candidal overgrowth in diabetic patients: potential predisposing factors. Mycoses. 2005;48(3):192- 6.

51. Adiaratou W hamed saleh. Epidemio-clinical aspects of lesions of the oral mucosa in 266 diabetic patients followed in hospital in Mali. [Mali]: Faculty of Medicine and Odontostomatology; 2019.

52. Mamari A, Hegami M, Sophiany N, Zom E, Heeded W, Atab R, et al. PREVALENCE OF ORAL CANDIDIASIS AMONG DIABETICS - NON DIABETICS PATIENTS AND EVALUATETHE CONTRIBUTION OF RISKFACTORS IN IBB CITY. Int J Adv Res. 31 Dec 2017;5(12):1372- 80.

53. Černáková L, Líšková A, Lengyelová L, Rodrigues CF. Prevalence and Antifungal Susceptibility Profile of Oral Candida spp. Isolates from a Hospital in Slovakia. Medicina (Mex). 22 Apr 2022;58(5):576.

54. Sharma U. Isolation and Speciation of Candida in Type II Diabetic Patients using CHROM Agar: A Microbial Study. J Clin Diagn Res [Internet]. 2017 [cited 29 May 2022]; Available from Available from: http://jcdr.net/article_fulltext.asp?issn=0973-709x&year=2017&volume=11&issue=8&page=DC09&issn=0973-709x&id=10394

55. Khosravi AR, Yarahmadi S, Baiat M, Shokri H, Pourkabireh M. Factors affecting the prevalence of yeasts in the oral cavity of patients with diabetes mellitus. J Mycol Médicale. 1 June 2008;18(2):83- 8.

56. Al Mubarak S, Robert AA, Baskaradoss JK, Al-Zoman K, Al Sohail A, Alsuwyed A, et al. The prevalence of oral Candida infections in periodontitis patients with type 2 diabetes mellitus. J Infect Public Health. August 2013;6(4):296- 301.

57. Vijay S, Bansal N, Rao BK, Veeraraghavan B, Rodrigues C, Wattal C, et al. Secondary Infections in Hospitalized COVID-19 Patients: Indian Experience. Infect Drug Resist. May 2021;Volume 14:1893- 903.

58. Salehi M, Ahmadikia K, Mahmoudi S, Kalantari S, Jamalimoghadamsiahkali S, Izadi A, et al. Oropharyngeal candidiasis in hospitalised COVID- 19 patients from Iran: Species identification and antifungal susceptibility pattern. Mycoses. August 2020;63(8):771- 8.

59. Duggal R, Goswami R, Xess I, Duggal I, Talwar A, Mathur VP. Prevalence of species-specific candidiasis and status of oral hygiene and dentition among diabetic patients: A hospital-based study. Indian J Dent Res. 7 Jan 2021;32(3):292.

GLOSSARY

Aspergillosis: is an opportunistic infection that usually affects the lower respiratory tract and is caused by inhalation of spores of the filamentous fungus aspergillus, commonly found in the environment.

Bruxism: defined as the involuntary grinding or clenching of teeth. It is a disorder that can affect both adults and children unconsciously. The severity and extent of bruxism can vary over the course of a lifetime.

Chloramphenicol: is a phenicol antibiotic used in combination with gentamicin in mycological culture media to inhibit bacterial growth.

Gram stain: this is the staining method most commonly used in medical bacteriology. It is used to colour bacteria and distinguish them on direct examination by their ability to bind gentian violet (gram +) or fuschin (gram -).

Grocott stain: used in histology to visualise fungi, certain pathogens, basal membranes and argentaffin histological structures in general.

PAS (periodic acid shiff) staining: is the most versatile and widely used technique for visualising carbohydrates.

Cycloheximide: is an antifungal agent that blocks protein biosynthesis in eukaryotic cells. It is also used in microbiology as a fungus growth inhibitor (antifungal) in the design of selective culture media.

Bacterial flora: all the micro-organisms living in a natural or pathological state in certain parts of the body.

Cornmeal agar: is a well-established mycological medium that is a suitable substrate for the production of chlamydospores by candida albicans and the maintenance of cultures of fungal strains.Gentamicin: is an antibiotic in the aminoglycoside family.
Giemsa: is a chromosome-specific dye, made up of a mixture of two dyes (methylene blue and eosin) in a purplish-pink colour, used in particular to highlight chromosome territories.
Gingivitis: inflammation of the gums, which become red, swollen and bleed.

Haematoxylin and eosin: are two dyes commonly used on tissue samples so that they can be seen under the microscope. Haematoxylin adheres to dna which turns the nucleus blue or purple. Eosin adheres to proteins and other parts cells, turning them pink or red.

Molecular hybridization: is a technique used to identify a nucleic acid sequence within a cell, tissue or particular environment. It is based on the principle of complementarity of nucleic bases, more specifically between complementary strands of DNA or RNA.

Insulin: a protein hormone, secreted in the pancreas by the islets of langerhans, which controls the concentration of glucose in the blood. Insulin deficiency leads to diabetes mellitus.

Periodontal disease: characterised by progressive gingival inflammation with destruction of the tissues supporting the teeth, i.e. the bone and alveolar ligaments, leading to tooth mobility which can lead to tooth loss.PCB medium: is an agar-based culture medium used to detect candida albicans chlamydospores.

Mucormycoses: are invasive infections caused by ubiquitous filamentous fungi belonging to the order Mucorales. They occur particularly in patients who are immunocompromised, diabetic or who have undergone organ transplants.

Neutrophils: are blood cells belonging to the white lineage. They are white blood cells (leukocytes) which play a major role in the immune system.

Lingual papillae: these are small growths that cover the tongue. Some of them contain taste buds which play a role in the perception of taste: these are the taste buds.

PCR (polymerase chain reaction) is an enzymatic amplification technique used to obtain a large number of identical copies of a DNA fragment.

Dental prosthesis: is a dental device that replaces one or more missing teeth and, if necessary, the associated anatomical structures.

Sarcoidosis: is an inflammatory disease characterized by infiltration of one or more lymph nodes. several organs and tissues by granulomas without caseous necrosis.
Cushing's syndrome: clinical abnormalities secondary chronic elevation of cortisol or other corticosteroids.

Acquired immunodeficiency syndrome AIDS: a set of symptoms resulting the destruction of immune system cells by the human immunodeficiency virus.

APPENDICES

Appendix 1: Information sheet

Nº de tube	Service	Type Diabète	Ancienneté Diabète	Diabète Equilibré ?	Mesure Hygiéno-diététique		Sexe	Age	Motif d'hospitalisation	Signe clinique	Antécédents médicaux et chirurgicaux	Traitement reçu	Durée d'hospitalisation	Espèce
					Brossage	Consultation dentiste								
01	P	I		OUI	OUI	OUI	H							
	C													
	T	II		NON	NON	NON	F							
	I													
02	P	I		OUI	OUI	OUI	H							
	C													
	T	II		NON	NON	NON	F							
	I													
03	P	I		OUI	OUI	OUI	H							
	C													
	T	II		NON	NON	NON	F							
	I													

Annex 2: Colorimetric Auxanogram

1. Clinical interest

Over the last decade, the number of yeast infections has increased dramatically, particularly in immunocompromised patients. Although Candida albicans is the most frequently isolated yeast from clinical samples, the emergence of non-albicans species has clearly been a recent concern.

On the other hand, the emergence of yeast species that are less sensitive to the new agents antifungal agents explains the importance of their rapid identification. The Auxacolor system has proved reliable when used in conjunction with morphological tests and is easy to use for identifying the most medically important yeasts.

2. Test principle

AUXACOLOR TM 2 is an identification system based on the assimilation of sugars. Yeast growth is visualised by turning a pH indicator.

3. How it works

- **Inoculation of the microplate**

Under sterile conditions, the suspension medium is inoculated with colonies of the pure strain a 24 to 48 h culture on Sabouraud medium supplemented with a sufficient quantity of chloramphenicol. After homogenising the suspension with a vortex, 100 µlthe inoculum is pipetted into each of the microplate wells Cover the microplate with an adhesive, making sure that the adhesion is perfectly uniform. Incubate for 48 hours (72 hours if necessary) at 27°C.

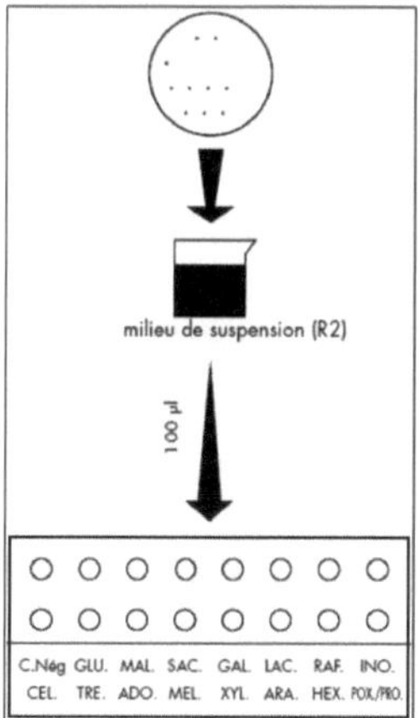

Figure 62. Schematic diagram of the Auxacolor procedure

- **Reading the results**

After 48 hours, when the yeast assimilates the sugars, it multiplies, resulting in a cloudiness in the cups. The change in colour observed helps interpret the positive and negative reactions, and a coding system is then established.The final identification of the species is based on a combination of biochemical tests and additional characteristics (morphological and metabolic) determined under the usual conditions.

Appendix 3: Strain interpretation table based on the results observed in the Auxacolor microplate

TABLEAU D'INTERPRETATION	GLU.	MAL.	SAC.	GAL.	LAC.	RAF.	INO.	CEL.	TRE.	ADO.	MEL.	XYL.	ARA.	HEX.	POX./PRO.		PL.	AR.	CA.	MY.	CHL.	37°C
SOUCHES																				PS -MY.		
C. ALBICANS 1	+	+	+	+	-	-	-	-	+ (-)	V	V	+ (-)	V	+ (-)	-	+	-	-	-	+	+ (-)	+
C. ALBICANS 2 [1]	+	+	-	+	-	-	-	-	V	V	-	V	V	+	-	-	-	-	-	+	+ (-)	+
C. CIFERRII	+	+	+	+	-	+ (-)	+	V	+	+	-	+	+	V	-	-	-	-	-	+	-	+
C. DUBLINIENSIS	+	+	+	+	-	-	-	-	V	+ (-)	- (+)	-	-	+ (-)	-	+	-	-	-	+	+	+
C. FAMATA	+	+	+	+	V	+	-	+	+	+	+ (-)	V	V	-	-	V	-	-	-	-	-	V
C. GLABRATA	+	-	-	-	- (+)	-	-	-	+	-	-	-	-	-	-	-	-	-	-	-	-	+
C. GUILLIERMONDII	+	+	+	+	-	+ (-)	-	+	+	+ (-)	+ (-)	+ (-)	+	-	-	+	-	-	-	+	-	+
C. INCONSPICUA	+	-	-	-	-	-	-	-	- (+)	-	-	-	-	-	-	V	-	-	-	-	-	+
C. KEFYR	+	-	+	+	+ (-)	+	-	V	- (+)	- (+)	-	V	V	-	-	-	-	-	-	+ (-)	-	+
C. KRUSEI	+	-	-	-	-	-	-	-	-	-	-	-	-	-	-	- (+)	-	-	-	+	-	+
C. LIPOLYTICA	+	-	-	- (+)	-	-	-	- (+)	-	- (+)	-	-	-	-	-	+ (-)	-	-	-	+	-	V
C. LUSITANIAE	+	+	+	+ (-)	- (+)	-	-	+	+	V	+	+ (-)	V	-	-	V	-	-	-	+ (-)	-	+
C. NORVEGENSIS	+	-	-	-	-	-	-	+ (-)	-	-	-	- (+)	-	-	-	+	-	-	-	+	-	+
C. PARAPSILOSIS	+	+	+	+	-	-	-	-	+ (-)	V	+ (-)	+ (-)	+	-	-	V	-	-	-	+	-	+
C. RUGOSA	+	-	-	+ (-)	-	-	-	-	-	V	-	V	- (+)	-	-	V	-	-	-	+	-	+
C. SAKE	+	+	+	V	-	-	-	V	+	V	+	V	-	+ (-)	-	V	-	-	-	+	-	-
C. TROPICALIS	+	+	+ (-)	+	-	-	-	V	+	+ (-)	+	+	-	-	-	- (+)	-	-	-	+	-	+
C. ZEYLANOIDES	+	-	-	- (+)	-	-	-	- (+)	+ (-)	V	-	-	-	- (+)	-	+ (-)	-	-	-	+	-	- (+)
C. ALBIDUS	+	+	+	V	V	V	V	+	V	V	+	+	V	-	-	V	-	-	+	-	-	V
C. LAURENTII	+	+	+	+	+	+	+	+	+	+	+	+	+	-	-	-	-	-	+	-	-	-
C. NEOFORMANS	+	+	+	+	-	V	+	V	V	V	+ (-)	V	V	-	+ (-)	-	-	-	+	-	-	+
C. UNIGUTTULATUS	+	+	+	V	-	V	+	-	V	V	+	+ (-)	V	-	-	V	-	-	+	-	-	-
G. CANDIDUM	+	-	-	+ (-)	-	-	-	-	-	V	-	+	-	-	- (+)	- (+)	-	+	-	+	-	- (+)
G. CAPITATUM	+	-	-	V	-	-	-	-	-	-	-	-	-	-	-	-	-	+	-	+	-	+
K. APICULATA	+	-	-	-	-	-	-	+	-	-	-	-	-	-	-	-	-	-	-	-	-	-
R. GLUTINIS	+	+	+	V	-	V	-	V	+	V	+	V	V	V	-	+	+	-	-	-	-	V
R. MUCILAGINOSA (RUBRA)	+	V	+	V	-	+	-	V	V	V	V	V	V	V	-	+	+	-	-	-	-	V
S. CEREVISIAE	+	+ (-)	+	V	-	+ (-)	-	-	V	-	V	-	-	-	-	-	-	-	-	- (+)	-	V
T. ASAHII	+	+	V	+	+	-	V	+	V	V	V	V	V	+ (-)	-	-	-	+	-	+	-	+
T. INKIN	+	+	+	V	+	-	+ (-)	+	+ (-)	-	+	+	V	+ (-)	-	-	-	+	-	+	-	+
T. MUCOIDES	+	+	+	+	+	+	+	+	+	+ (-)	+	+	+	V	-	-	-	+	-	+	-	+
T. SPP	+	+	+ (-)	+ (-)	+	V	V	+	+ (-)	V	V	+ (-)	+ (-)	V	-	- (+)	-	+	-	+	-	V
P. WICKERHAMII [2]	+	-	-	+ (-)	V	-	-	-	+	-	-	-	-	-	-	-	-	-	-	-	-	+

SUMMARY

Introduction

Oral candidiasis is a disease of the oral cavity caused by yeasts of the genus Candida, which develops in patients with a fragile immune system, particularly immunocompromised patients, including diabetics. We conducted a prospective descriptive study at the Batna University Hospital. The main objective of our study was to determine the prevalence of oral candidiasis in diabetic patients hospitalised in the various departments at Batna University Hospital, and to describe the risk factors and the species involved.

Materials and methods

We included 78 diabetic patients in our study. Mouth swabs using sterile swabs were taken from each patient and an information was filled in, including demographic, clinical, therapeutic and biological data. The samples were cultured. Candida species were identified using the Auxacolor kit.

Results

The prevalence of oral candidiasis in our study was 63%. Males predominated (53%). The majority of patients were hospitalised in the paediatric ward, with a frequency of 40%, and the most common species was Candida albicans. The main risk factors contributing to the occurrence of this disease were antibiotic therapy, diabetic ketoacidosis and the wearing dental prostheses.

Conclusion

Systemic health is linked to oral health, particularly in people with diabetes, which requires rigorous management and the involvement of healthcare professionals in strategies for recognising, preventing and screening for this disease. The inclusion of an oral examination for diabetic patients has therefore become essential.

***Key words**: Candida, oral candidiasis, diabetes, oral cavity.*

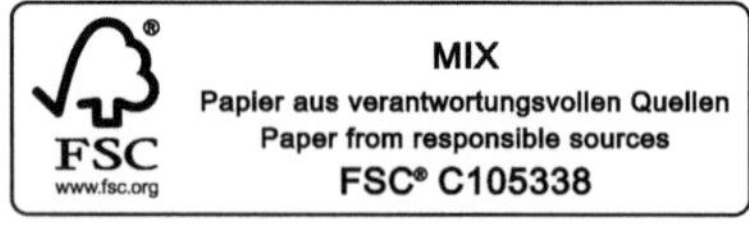

Printed by Books on Demand GmbH, Norderstedt / Germany